IronFit®
Triathlon Training
for Women

IronFit®

Triathlon Training for Women

Training Programs and Secrets
for Success in all Triathlon Distances

Melanie Fink and Don Fink

Guilford, Connecticut

To our service women and men who defend our freedom
and allow us the liberty to pursue our dreams.

CONTENTS

Introduction

Female participation in the sport of triathlon has skyrocketed worldwide since the year 2000. What's even more amazing than this phenomenal growth is the fact that the ratio of women in the sport has greatly increased during this same time frame. Women are now the most rapidly growing segment in one of the world's fastest-growing sports.

In no place is this more apparent than in the United States. Membership in USA Triathlon, the governing body of the sport in the United States, has more than quadrupled in the past twelve years, climbing from about 127 thousand members in 2000 to over 550 thousand members today. As amazing as this growth is, even more amazing is the fact that women make up the fastest-growing segment of this rapidly growing sport. While women accounted for only about 25 percent of the USA Triathlon membership in the year 2000, their participation has skyrocketed to about 40 percent today. And these statistics are only for the United States—there are now millions of women competing in triathlon worldwide.

Along with the amazing growth in the participation of female triathletes has been a growth in their competitiveness. Women want to do a lot more than just participate—they want to compete, and their race times have been getting progressively faster each year. Today, competitions in the female age groups are as fiercely battled as any of the men's age groups.

This has resulted in a hunger for information specific to female triathletes. The challenge for women, however, is that while they encounter all the same challenges as men, a host of additional issues exist that are unique to them . . . most of which men don't have a clue about. From the stay-at-home mom to the professional woman, female triathletes face a wide range of challenges including societal expectations and physical and emotional issues. Until now, there has been no single go-to source for this type of information and guidance.

This book provides exactly what the fastest-growing segment of the triathlon world yearns for: a complete training guide for female triathletes with highly efficient and easy-to-follow training programs for success in all triathlon distances. It is geared toward women of all experience and competitive levels, from the beginner to the seasoned veteran triathlete. This book arms the female triathlete with everything she needs to know to persevere over these unique challenges, and it provides her with the exact step-by-step training programs to help her to achieve her goals and more.

We have been training female athletes for over twenty years and have enjoyed success at all levels. From being the first overall woman at a regional triathlon to winning their age groups at the Ironman World Championships in Kona, Hawaii, IronFit's female athletes have been a force. And more important, IronFit has successfully inspired and brought women into the sport through our time-efficient approach and practical training plans. Through this book we share the training secrets and training plans guaranteed to help any female triathlete take her performance to the next level.

We will start by presenting the illustrious history of women in triathlon. This may be surprising to some, as most women are not even aware of the crucial role women have played in the successful growth of the sport from the very beginning.

Then we will present successful training and lifestyle strategies for you as a female triathlete and discuss the important health and nutritional challenges affecting women. We deal with all of the physical and emotional issues confronting women, some of which are sensitive and rarely discussed. But it is important information that female athletes need to know.

We will then provide all the information needed to empower you to select the best races and to set highly motivating goals. The criteria for selecting races and setting exciting and healthy goals for women often differ from that of men, and we address those issues head on.

Next we will provide advice on triathlon equipment for women. Should you use equipment specifically designed for women or the same equipment the men use? It actually depends on the type of equipment, and we will spell it all out for you.

We will fully explain all of the specific training sessions that make up a great training program, as well as the crucial training principles for success, and we will show you the secrets of making "heart rate" training work for you.

This book includes three complete multileveled training programs specially designed for women at the Sprint/Standard (aka "Olympic") Distance, Half Iron-Distance, and Full Iron-Distance triathlons. Each program is presented at three levels: Competitive, Intermediate, and Just-Finish. You can simply select the program for the race distance for which you want to train and the exact level, based on your individual competitiveness, experience, and available training time. The proper training program, combined with the information presented in this book, will provide you with everything you need to successfully prepare for and maximize your performance at any racing distance.

In addition to the actual training programs, we will present our Functional Strength and Core Program, Warm-Up Program, and Flexibility Program, all specifically designed for female triathletes.

Next, we cover proper techniques in swimming, cycling, and running and provide tools for improving and fine-tuning your form. We will discuss transitions (T1 and T2), which is often referred to as the "fourth sport" of triathlon, and we will provide tips and strategies for becoming faster and more efficient in T1 and T2. Finally, we present specific training programs and guidance on exactly what you should do in the "off-season" to best prepare for the next season and to ensure continued improvement year after year, as well as how to bridge the gap between races.

As with all of our books, this book is not written in a highly technical and complicated manner. Instead, we present direct information and training programs in an easy-to-understand and enjoyable way while addressing the issues and obstacles that women face. After reading this book you can immediately put the information to work and get right on the road to accomplishing your triathlon dreams.

Throughout the book we will include profiles of successful and inspiring female triathletes. These accounts will be motivational, and you are likely to relate to and see yourself in many of these athletes. These profiles will demonstrate how the goal is achievable, how obstacles can be overcome, and how you can keep your family life and career in balance. You will see how the journey can be even more rewarding than first imagined.

As complicated and challenging as the road to success in triathlon can be for anyone, it's even more complicated and challenging for women. Many more factors and issues must be taken into account. This book provides the female triathlete with a truly unique and all-encompassing road map to success.

One more important point we always like to remind our coached athletes of: It's going to be *fun*! There is a reason triathlon is growing so rapidly, and it's the same reason that the ratio of women within triathlon is growing even faster, and that reason is simply that it's fun. It's about enjoying the challenge and enjoying the journey. This will surely be one of your most enjoyable and rewarding adventures ever, from start to finish.

So, let's now turn the page and begin this amazing journey together!

CHAPTER 1

The Amazing History of Women in Triathlon

I'm building a fire, and every day I train, I
add more fuel. At just the right moment, I
light the match.

— *Mia Hamm, Olympic gold medal soccer player*

By reading this book, you are already part of the illustrious history of women in the sport of triathlon. If you are new to the sport, you will surely be surprised at the crucial role women have played in the founding and success of triathlon. As you will see, it can even be argued that women have played a more significant role in the growth and popularity of the sport than men. Most important, this rich history of women in triathlon continues to inspire and motivate new generations of triathletes today.

Most triathlon historians agree that the first triathlon of modern times was the Mission Bay race hosted by members of the San Diego Track Club in September of 1974. Women were among the seventy-four athletes who participated in that very first race. How many popular sports exist today for which you can claim that women participated in the very first event?

Flash-forward to 1979, the second year of the Hawaii Ironman, the most important and famous of all triathlons. Champion cyclist Lyn Lemaire became the world's first female Ironman when she finished fifth overall against her male competitors. Lyn held the US 40-kilometer cycling time trial record at the time and had been a standout high school swimmer. She courageously brought her talents to Hawaii in the late 1970s and became one of the true pioneers in the sport of triathlon.

We often have to laugh when some uninformed person asks us if women race the same distance as the men in triathlon. It seems like a crazy question—of course they do—but when you consider a sport like professional

1

tennis where women actually play fewer sets than the men do, we guess it is not such a crazy question. But women sure *do* race the same distance as the men. Every woman has, from Lyn Lemaire to the thousands and thousands of women since. Maybe that works for tennis, but not our sport. Never has, never will.

Let's now jump ahead to 1982 and what is generally considered to be the single most significant event in the history and global growth of triathlon. And guess what! It involved just two women.

A graduate student from California named Julie Moss found herself leading the Hawaii Ironman late into the run. An international audience watched the event on *ABC's Wide World of Sports* and became glued to their televisions as she started to show signs of dehydration. First she started to wobble ... then she stumbled ... then she righted herself and continued on ... only to stumble again. With over 140 miles completed and less than 10 yards to the finish line, she found that all she could do was crawl on her hands and knees.

The athletic world held their collective breath watching her epic struggle. Then, as race officials and spectators walked alongside the crawling athlete cheering her on to complete those last few yards, fellow American Kathleen McCartney Hearst ran past her for the victory. It was both spellbinding and

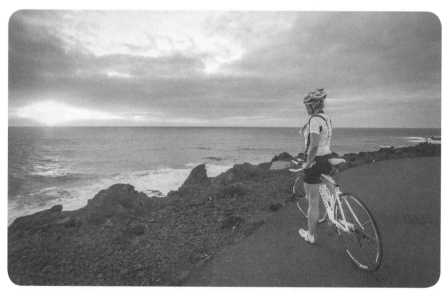

Pro triathlete and national record holder Aya Stevens / *James Mitchell Photography*

extraordinary. The sight of Julie Moss crawling to the finish line only to be passed by Kathleen McCartney became synonymous with *ABC's Wide World of Sports's* famous tag line: "The thrill of victory and the agony of defeat."

And like nothing before or after it, this one single event launched an upstart sport into the global consciousness. The sport has never been the same since, and it can all be traced back to these two female athletes in 1982. This emotional and extraordinary spectacle, viewed by millions, was the single-biggest event to ignite the explosion in popularity that triathlon enjoys today.

Eighteen years later triathlon became an official Olympic sport and debuted as the kickoff event at the 2000 Summer Olympics in Sydney, Australia. An equal number of women and men competed for gold, silver, and bronze. This may not seem like a significant point to make, but when you compare this to other sports, you can see how truly meaningful it is.

The modern Olympics began in the year 1896. The men's marathon was part of the games that year and in every Olympics since. But amazingly, women were not allowed to run the marathon in the Olympics until the Los Angeles games in 1984. That's right: It took some eighty-eight years for the Olympics to include the women's marathon. This fact, combined with the other events we have mentioned above, demonstrate how truly special the sport of triathlon is and the vital role women have played in the sport's incredible growth and success.

Today millions of women compete worldwide in the sport and the only thing faster than the growth of triathlon today appears to be the growth of female participation within triathlon. Twelve years ago women comprised only about 25 percent of triathlon participation in North America. Today that number is about 40 percent. And that is just for the United States. There are millions of women competing worldwide in triathlon today.

While we consider Lyn Lemaire, Julie Moss, and Kathleen McCartney Hearst to be some of the greatest pioneers of triathlon, following in their footsteps was a series of female stars that inspired generations of new triathletes. While there is a long list of female triathlon stars who fit this description, there are two additional Ironman Hall of Fame inductees we would like to specifically cite: Karen Smyers and Paula Newby Fraser.

American Karen Smyers became a dominant figure in the sport in the 1990s. While her list of accomplishments is too long to cover, some of her career highlights include winning three ITU World titles, seven national titles, and one Ironman World Championship title, and as a member of the 2000 USA Olympic team, she was selected to carry her nation's colors in Sydney. Amazingly, Karen is a cancer survivor, a mother of two, and today in her fifties, continues to actively race at a high level. Her perseverance, sense of humor, and tenacity have made her a true ambassador of our sport and an inspiration to all.

Paula Newby Fraser, originally from South Africa and Zimbabwe, established herself as one of the most dominant Iron-distance competitors ever. A nationally ranked swimmer as a child, she took up triathlon in the 1980s and between the years 1986 and 1996 won eight Ironman World titles, earning her the nickname "The Queen of Kona." Paula also became the first woman ever to break nine hours for the Ironman distance and finished as high as eleventh overall among the men in some very competitive years. *Triathlete* magazine has declared her "the Greatest Triathlete in History" and ABC Sports and the *Los Angeles Times* have declared her "the Greatest All-Round Female Athlete in the World." When it comes to Iron-distance racing, the Queen of Kona has set the standard for all those who come after her to be measured against.

One of the most significant phenomena in the history and growth of women in triathlon was the emergence of women-only races. These races made triathlon accessible to tens of thousands of women who may not have entered the sport if racing with men were the only option. The Danskin triathlon, which was started in 1990, claims to have hosted over 130 races and over 250,000 female athletes over a twenty-year period. Under the wise guidance of another great triathlon pioneer, Sally Edwards, the Danskin series went out of its way to ensure a very comfortable and welcoming environment for new women entering the sport. There are surely thousands of women today who may never have tried a triathlon had it not been for Sally Edwards and the Danskin triathlon series.

In addition to what women-only races provide for women athletes, they also provide a wonderful marketing opportunity for companies with products and services targeted at this attractive market. From a business standpoint, it can be a perfect fit. In fact, the explosion of the number of women in the sport has led to successful new industries and product lines to support the growing need for women-specific triathlon equipment and training and racing clothing.

Today there are spectacular women-only races and women-only race series across North America. One of our favorites is the Iron Girl Triathlon series, which started with two events in 2004 and now has nineteen across the United States, plus three more international races. This series offers prize money and many of the series' races, like the Iron Girl Columbia Triathlon in Maryland, regularly draw over 2,000 participants.

Other popular women-only triathlon series include Esprit de She, Mermaid Triathlon & Duathlon, Girls Gone Tri, Rocket Chix, and many more. And those are only the series—there are countless independent woman-only races as well, including the Tri Goddess Triathlon in Michigan, the Girl Power Triathlon in Louisiana, and the Jersey Girl Triathlon in—you guessed it—New Jersey.

A recent check of trifind.com, a popular online race calendar, lists more than 200 women-only races just in the United States. In Appendix C we have included links to some of our favorites.

The phenomenon of women-only races has been another crucial part of the illustrious history of women in triathlon. And after only about four decades since those first brave women participated in that first triathlon at Mission Bay, the story has only begun to be written.

Where will women's triathlon go from here? The sky's the limit and only the future will tell. Certainly part of the future story will come from the college ranks. In January 2014 we had yet another watershed moment for women's triathlon. The National Collegiate Athletic Association (NCAA) in the United States approved women's triathlon as a Division I, II, and III college sport. This virtually ensures that the phenomenal growth of women's triathlon will continue for generations to come.

Unlike most other sports, women have been part of triathlon from the very beginning. What's more, they have played an equal, if not more significant, role in the sport's amazing success and growth since the 1970s. All signs indicate that women are positioned to continue this trend far into the future.

The future of triathlon is bright, and the future of women in this sport is even brighter. And if you are reading this book, you are likely going to be part of that bright future.

Following is our first of seven motivating profiles of an inspiring female triathlete.

ATHLETE SUCCESS STORY:
BETH POORE

While reading a women's health magazine over ten years ago, Beth Poore came across an advertisement for the women-only Danskin Sprint Triathlon Series organized by triathlon great Sally Edwards. Along with the race details was Danskin's motto, "The woman who starts the race is not the same woman who finishes the race." Although she competed in sports all her life, Beth could not recall ever feeling *transformed* at a sporting event's conclusion, even after completing a marathon. This intrigued her so much that she signed up for her first triathlon.

Beth not only successfully completed her first triathlon, she loved the entire experience and the triathlon environment. And like so many other women who tried a Danskin series race, she became hooked on triathlon.

Now over ten years later, Beth has completed more than fifteen triathlons, including four Iron-Distance triathlons, in addition to a countless number of road races. The amazing thing about Beth is that she has continually improved her performances year after year and consistently lowers her racing times. When we asked what she considers the accomplishment of which she is most proud, Beth said, "Sustainability in the sport. Making incremental improvements each year, and balancing the three-legged stool: family, career, and triathlon."

Beth Poore's advice for women entering triathlon: "1) Set manageable goals, which build confidence and a strong foundation; 2) follow a good training plan or consider hiring an experienced coach; 3) be flexible in training and on race day . . . expect the unexpected; 4) define your training strategy, e.g., alone, with a friend, with a group; 5) find a triathlon mentor or someone who can answer questions and be a sounding board; 6) be patient—improvement is built on cumulative effort; and 7) have fun!"

CHAPTER 2

Successful Training and Lifestyle Strategies for the Female Triathlete

Mental will is a muscle that needs exercise,
just like the muscles of the body.

—Lynn Jennings, world-class runner

To be successful in triathlon you must overcome many barriers and hurdles along the way. These can include your lifestyle choices and the many biases of being a woman. The challenges we face in attempting to accomplish our triathlon goals, which some might consider selfish, can be overwhelming. You, as an athlete and more so as a woman, face not only the physical and time factors but also the societal pressures of being a woman, from the "stay-at-home" mom to the working woman.

You have a unique set of challenges to overcome when embarking toward the goal of becoming a triathlete and competing regularly in triathlon. Women we coach often say things like "I feel guilty getting a babysitter so I can train" or "I work full-time and I feel guilty leaving my family to go out and train when I get home." Or even, "How am I going to tell my boss I have to leave the office by 6:30 p.m. to make it to my Masters Swim class?" These are questions you have probably asked yourself at one point or another and can probably add many more to the list.

Aside from those legitimate challenges, another real challenge that women face is general safety issues in their training. Running and riding alone can be very dangerous for anyone, but it can be especially unsafe for women. We know it can be difficult to coordinate your schedule with a friend or training group, and oftentimes you have to train alone. This can be concerning, and we will share with you some safety practices you can put into place.

Although these are just some of the examples of the challenges women face, we have pretty much heard them all. And we both empathize and sympathize with your situation, but don't be dismayed: It can and has been done quite successfully by many women all over the world. And by women of all shapes, sizes, and financial backgrounds, single, married, with or without children, working or studying. And for you first-timers about to embark on your triathlon journey, you can and *will* do it too.

So, what are some of the issues and hurdles that female athletes face in their daily lives? Let's take a look at those most prevalent today and some of the strategies to deal with them.

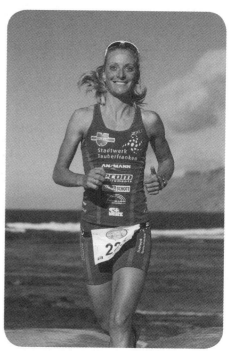

Pro triathlete and Ironman champion Heidi Sessner / *James Mitchell Photography*

Societal Pressures and Biases of the Female Role

Although fading quite rapidly here in the United States, the old biases of the female role in society still face us today. Some of you will face resistance from older-generation family members who think you should be devoted to your husband and children 100 percent of the time, while some of you may simply experience the stereotypical gender bias from both men and other women. This can not only create tension and friction between family members, it can also create an unsupportive environment and sometimes lead to sabotaging your efforts.

As time goes on, these biases too will fade. But for now we have to learn to deal with them. So, although the family meeting described below might be helpful in a lot of situations, it may not be useful in certain situations. We have worked with athletes who just keep their training and racing to their immediate family (spouse and children) and those athletes who actually end up estranging family members over it. This, of course, is a worst-case scenario, but it does happen.

Here are some successful approaches to overcoming some of these biases and misperceptions:

- **Drag them along:** We have found a strategy that often works is to bring those family members to a race to experience the positive buzz of the event and get inspired. Sometimes, once a family member attends one of your races, it spurs a very proud moment for him and actually has the opposite effect than you thought it would. Family members see many women doing the same thing with supportive spouses and family, and it makes them want to support your efforts and help out more.
- **Keep it to yourself:** We know from many of our athletes that oftentimes family members, friends, and neighbors are just not that interested in your extracurricular activities. So rather than forcing your lifestyle or sharing your experiences with them, just "keep it to yourself" around those folks.
- **Birds of a feather:** Befriend other women triathletes with whom you can train or connect over coffee to share your experiences. Finding friends who share your interests and understand your motivation can be helpful in satisfying your need to talk about your triathlon training and racing with someone who is supportive and empathetic.
- **Role models:** Surround yourself with positive people in the sport and look to women who have done it already and can give you support as you head out on your journey. Connect through social media and garner their insights and wisdom to help you through the many challenges you will face along the way.
- **Be a "happy warrior":** You need to make a conscious decision up front about how you will handle the situation of unsupportive family and friends and put a plan in place to deal with it. Then be the happy warrior and leave it at that. Hopefully, your spouse or partner is supportive enough, and that is all you will need to accomplish your goals and live the lifestyle you have chosen. It is all about the journey, and you want that journey to begin on a positive note.

There are many challenges you face as a woman in the sport, so let's look at some specific situations that may help you if you fall into one of these categories. However, even if you don't, these strategies may be applied across the board and all women can benefit from them. Having worked with so many female athletes with varying family, work, and school situations, here are some examples of strategies that our athletes have shared with us that have proven extremely successful.

The Stay-at-Home Mom

The stay-at-home mom has her unique issues. Here are some great strategies to help you navigate your way to becoming a successful and happy triathlete:

- **The "mom shift":** It is about scheduling your training around your children's schooling and other activities. Weekends are the highest-volume training days for the programs in this book because this works the best for athletes with Monday-to-Friday jobs. But this may not be the case for most moms, who often have less time to train on the weekend because of various family activities. Many of these athletes will take the training programs in this book and shift them ahead three or four days, while keeping everything in order. This allows them to have the busiest training days during the week and their lighter training days on the weekends.
- **"The family train":** It is about including your children in your training. For instance, set up your bike trainer in the kids' playroom while they are doing homework or other activities. Or if your children are old enough, include them in your run by riding their bikes next to you. One of our coached athletes, Mo Cullen, often has her children set up to do activities while she is on her trainer and finds it a most effective way to meet the many demands of being a stay-at-home mom. Another coached athlete, Judi Germano, often has her son and daughter ride their bikes next to her during her runs.
- **Carpooling:** You probably do some of this already, but make it a regular weekly schedule and use that time to make training more consistent and manageable and less of a disruption to the family. Arrange carpooling with your training buddies or neighbors a few

times a week, so you can fit in a morning workout and avoid unforeseen issues that might come up later in the day, like a sick child.

Professional Women and Working Moms

For those women who work full-time, outside the home, with or without children, your challenges can be just as complicated. And for any women in high school or college, you too can use these strategies to help you fit in your training. In the morning you may have to get the kids up and off to school, leaving little time to train before work. Or you may have to catch an early train to get to work or school. Here are some helpful strategies you might want to consider:

- **Early-morning training:** Consider getting up before everyone else and fitting in a 30- to 60-minute workout before the morning preparation for the kids begins or before you have to leave for work or school. We know this is hard to do. However, the beauty of a morning workout is that you get it behind you first thing and it allows you to focus on the rest of your day. And how many times have you said, "Oh, I will workout tonight when I get home," and then you get home late and are too tired to muster the strength to go to the gym, right? It happens to all of us so do what you can to minimize those occurrences.
- **Indoor training:** There are times during the year when it is difficult to get outside, or if you workout in the early morning or late evening, it is too dark. If this is your only option, then you have to embrace indoor training. There are many ways to mix it up and that includes using various cardio equipment to doing circuit training. Another convenience is that it is much easier to prepare your workout clothing in advance and have it ready because you know you will be indoors.
- **Lunchtime workouts:** This can be difficult given the time constraint of a one-hour lunch. Yes, "it's all about the hair!" as we hear so many of our female athletes complain. Getting the workout in and showering and drying hair is almost impossible to get done in an hour. Consider doing strength training for 30 minutes and forgo "washing the hair." Just make sure you don't have any afternoon appointments that you need to look your best for!
- **"On the way home" workouts:** Pack your bag in advance and be prepared to fit in a workout on your way home from work or school. It

is more likely you will get it done if you avoid stopping at home first. Then avoid the extra time away by showering when you get home.

- **Spin class:** You may want to ride your own bike, but that's not always an option when your time is limited. To get yourself motivated and have a little fun, hook up with a regular spin class in the early morning, at lunchtime, or after work to avoid the time-consuming complications of going out for a bike ride. If you ride outside, you understand the extra time it takes to get prepared for an outdoor ride, and this is a simple solution.
- **Train at your kid's game:** Where possible, consider running or riding to your child's event (e.g., soccer, lacrosse, baseball, etc.) or bring your bike trainer and set it up on the side of the field or parking lot so you can watch the game. It's an efficient way to kill two birds with one stone.
- **"Do what you can do now":** This is one of our favorite quotes by the great Dave Scott, six-time Hawaii Ironman World Champion. He used this quote in reference to racing, but it is so applicable to our training as well. For instance, let's say you have an hour-long run planned but you only have 30 minutes—do the 30 minutes. Avoid the trap of not doing anything or thinking you will have time later on to fit in the full 60 minutes . . . we know how that goes. Something comes up and you end up not fitting in a workout at all. Getting *something* done is better than nothing.
- **The "what-if" scenario:** It is best to think ahead about what can possibly go wrong and try to eliminate the risk before it happens. What if the babysitter gets sick or your boss wants you to stay late or the train is running late? These are all things that can cause you to miss a workout. An approach like getting your workouts done first thing in the morning is a great strategy to avoid this scenario. For those unavoidable other times, you just have to do your best. Avoid beating yourself up— just skip the workout and get right back on schedule the next day.

Safety Strategies

Some of the biggest concerns we hear from our female athletes are safety issues arising from training alone, either out on the bike or running on the roads very early in the morning or late at night. We hear many stories of women getting in bike accidents, getting injured while running, or just being caught in an unsafe area or situation. For many women, you know what we are talking about. You were riding your bike alone and some car pulls alongside of you with a bunch of guys in it and you can get uncomfortable very quickly. Here are some great ways to combat safety issues when training alone and avoiding those unsafe scenarios:

- **Pepper spray:** If you do not have pepper spray, we encourage you to get some today. Go to your local hardware store and pick up a key-ring or pocket-size pepper spray to carry with you when training outdoors. It can be used to scare off a stray animal while running or fend off a stranger if need be.
- **Cell phone:** Most everyone has one and you should by all means carry it with you when you train outdoors away from home. We do not recommend using it to text or make calls while you are running or biking, but certainly, having it available for an emergency is a necessity.
- **Road ID/credit card/cash:** Always carry some form of identification with you when you run or ride, along with a small amount of cash and/ or a credit card. You never know when you are going to need to buy something to get you home or get your bike repaired. A good company we like to recommend is Road ID (roadid.com). They have many forms of ID that you can use while running or biking.
- **Planned route/map:** We recommend you always leave a note when you leave the house or your dorm room with your planned bike or run route, even if you are only planning to go a few miles. It is better to be cautious and let others know your plan in case you run into trouble. This is especially true for women training on college campuses, in city parks, or in other wooded parks and hiking trails where unexpected things can happen.
- **Group training:** Although it is not always ideal given the varying abilities of athletes, it is a very smart and safe strategy to avoid training alone. You can hook up with a cycling group out of your local bike shop or triathlon club. There are running clubs in almost every city and town with runners at all abilities that you could connect with so you are not running alone. And when practicing your open-water swimming, it is a

must that you swim with a buddy. It is never a wise idea to swim alone in open water in any circumstance.

The Family Meeting

An approach for all women to consider is to have a family/friend meeting just as you embark toward your triathlon goals. It's always easiest when you have this meeting to talk about your goals and how important they are to you. Also discuss how you plan to make it as undisruptive as possible to everyone involved in achieving your goals. As helpful as it is to have a family meeting with your real family, it's also important to have one with your "work family" and anyone else who regularly relies on you. For example, schedule your workouts such that a coworker does not book a meeting with you at that time. Discuss with your husband or partner how you can share child care so you can both fit in your workouts or activities.

From our experience, we find spouses and partners to be very supportive of their significant others in triathlon. They are often agreeable to taking on child-care responsibilities to allow their partners to work out in the early morning or on the weekends. And it seems to work best when the partner reciprocates in kind. It makes for a happier relationship and a more calm family life. And it also sets a positive example for children.

We hope you find our suggestions, strategies, and tips in dealing with the lifestyle challenges that we all face useful in making triathlon a very satisfying and rewarding part of your life.

Following is the second of seven motivating profiles of an inspiring female triathlete.

ATHLETE SUCCESS STORY:
BREENA FISHBACK

Breena Fishback is married with two children and is a stay-at-home mom. She has been racing triathlon for over four years and has completed more than twelve races—her favorite being the Half Iron-Distance.

When we asked Breena which of her triathlon accomplishments she is most proud of, she simply said, "Getting started!" This is such a profound response. The first step in any great journey is usually the most important one. The first step is the one that breaks inertia and it's the one that takes true courage.

Sure, Breena had successfully competed in marathons and other road races, but triathlon was something totally different. For most, deciding to do a triathlon is an intimidating goal. But Breena not only decided to do a triathlon, she decided to do it on her own. She purchased the necessary equipment, she learned how to use it, she hired a coach, she signed up for a local race, and on the day before, she drove herself to the race packet pickup. She did it her way and she took control of the entire process. This truly is an accomplishment to be proud of.

Breena says that her greatest challenge in triathlon is balancing her family and home life responsibilities with her training and racing. She says that it is, "one thing to plug your training plan into your calendar, but it's another thing to stick to it when things like the weather, sick kids, vacation plans, etc., get in the way. Being flexible and planning ahead as much as possible are key. If there are poor road conditions one day, be willing and prepared to train indoors. If it cannot be done one day, use your 'slide days' to make sure that you can do it another day." (**Note:** We will discuss slide days in Chapter 6.)

Breena's advice for women considering triathlon is to "Carve out the time in your day/week/month to train and be a part of something extraordinary. If possible, find other women whose company you enjoy enough to train with. Hours and hours on a bike or running are much more enjoyable if there are a few people who can join you. But most of all enjoy the journey. Each training day and each race will bring its own challenges. Embrace them as best you can and keep putting one foot in front of the other. And finally, if possible, hire a great coach. Their expertise is worth its weight in gold!"

CHAPTER 3

Nutrition for Training, Racing, and a Healthy Lifestyle

The question isn't who is going to let me;
it's who is going to stop me.

—*Ayn Rand, novelist and philosopher*

As a female athlete, you want to eat healthfully and enjoy a healthy lifestyle as you pursue your triathlon goals. It is important to recognize that maintaining a healthy weight and supporting your training and racing requires a level of knowledge about nutrition and energy expenditure. For some this is a simple task; for others it is a constant struggle. Many of us will go through ups and downs with our nutrition and weight, and that's to be expected. We have times when we are very focused on it, like during our racing season, and other times we relax our attention to it.

It seems triathletes are always game for the latest and greatest nutritional trend out there, from chia seeds and coconut water to embracing the Paleo diet. There is always someone pitching the newest diet or nutrition fad out there, especially in the sport of triathlon. And that is all fine, but often we are deluged with so much information it causes more confusion than help.

So, how do we go about finding the right formula for us and applying it to our daily lives and training? We always like to recommend a common-sense approach and simple principles that you can apply to your life, no matter what your goals are.

Let's start with a few of the concepts that we use with our coached athletes and you can use while training and racing:

- **Grazing concept:** As an athlete, you want to maintain a consistent level of energy throughout the day to support a morning, afternoon, or evening workout. To do that, you might want to consider planning to

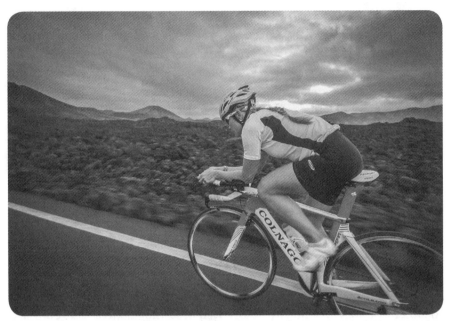

Pro triathlete and national record holder Aya Stevens / *James Mitchell Photography*

eat six smaller meals a day instead of three larger meals. Having smaller meals, or grazing, throughout the day helps you avoid highs and lows of energy and helps to prepare you better before and after a workout.

- **Balanced diet:** Too much of anything isn't a good thing. We encourage our athletes to have a balance of carbohydrates, fat, and protein at every meal. For most athletes, the 40/30/30 ratio (carbohydrates, fats, and protein) is a good starting point; then modify from there as you experiment.
- **Natural foods:** It's generally best to avoid processed foods as they are often filled with high sugar, fat, carbs, and sodium and oftentimes make you even hungrier than before you ate them. Think fresh foods like fruits, vegetables, whole grains, and nuts to get your daily dose of fiber and other nutrients. If you are gluten-free, you will find many foods like rice, quinoa, or other non-wheat-based natural foods that you can rely on. Almost every grocery store today has a gluten-free aisle.
- **Healthy snacks:** As part of the grazing concept, you want to make sure you incorporate healthy eating in between meals and possibly before

and after a workout, from a homemade shake with yogurt and berries or greens to a fresh piece of fruit or veggies with natural almond or peanut butter. These are the types of balanced snacks to incorporate into your everyday eating.

- **Supplements:** Generally our coached athletes will take a daily supplement including vitamins C and D, calcium, and magnesium that can help to keep them healthy in training. We recommend, though, that you have regular annual blood tests to determine if you have any vitamin deficiency before you begin a vitamin regimen. As described in Chapter 15 ("Health Strategies and Injury Prevention"), most women may want to take extra vitamins throughout their menstrual cycle or during menopause.

Optimizing Weight for Training and Racing

More often than not, our athletes are concerned with their weight and want to either lose weight generally or lose weight leading up to a race. For most women this is not an easy task. Combining dieting with training can be a bit more complicated than a simple diet alone. And for those few women who have the opposite issue of gaining or maintaining weight, you too will be able to follow these general guidelines to get you to your ideal weight.

A good rule of thumb for most athletes is the "5-pound off-season" guideline. You want to avoid putting on any more than 5 pounds in the off-season. From our experience, losing weight for women becomes more difficult as we age, so you want to stay within that 5-pound range (under or over). Otherwise, you can potentially risk injury when you start to increase volume and it can cause frustration, as it may take longer for you to return to your ideal fitness level. How do we go about figuring out our ideal weight for training and racing?

Body Mass Index (BMI)

Let's start by determining our optimal weight and some simple approaches to get there. You can use a number of sources to determine your optimal weight, but a good starting point is the body mass index, more widely known as your BMI. The formula to calculate your BMI is as follows:

Body mass index = weight (kg) / [height (m)]² (metric formula)
Weight (lbs.) / [Height (in.)]² x 703 (pounds formula)

This is a calculation to determine your health relative to your height and weight.

Unless you are a super mathematician, or you just enjoy solving complicated formulas like this, please consider using one of the many easy online BMI calculators like bmicalculator.org. All you need to input is your height, weight, and gender, and it does the calculation for you.

So, does BMI have its flaws? Yes. But again, it is a starting point. If your current BMI is in the healthy range of 18.5 to 24.9, you are presumably at a healthy weight. But the BMI calculation does not take into account your lean and fat body mass, which can be high for larger-boned women or more muscular women. If you are unsure, seek the advice of your doctor or certified nutritionist and share with her your athletic goals. To help us understand BMI, let's take a look at an example:

Tracy Triathlete is 5' 5" and weighs 145 lbs.
BMI = 145 lbs. / (65 inches)² x 703 = 24.13
Weight status: She is within the 18.5-to-24.9 normal range

HEIGHT	WEIGHT RANGE	BMI	WEIGHT STATUS
5' 5"	111 lbs. or less	Below 18.5	Underweight
	111 lbs. to 149 lbs.	18.5 to 24.9	Normal
	150 lbs. to 179 lbs.	25.0 to 29.9	Overweight
	180 lbs. or more	30 or higher	Obese

Using her current statistics, Tracy Triathlete ends up with a calculated BMI of 24.13. This falls within the normal range for the given standards of BMI. While this is a good place to start, most successful endurance athletes have a BMI in the lower half of the normal range. So, even though she has a normal BMI, Tracy may want to consider reducing her weight gradually over time to 130 pounds (or less), the midpoint of the normal range.

So, now that we know what we want our ideal weight to be, how do we get there? We like to go back to basics and use a daily calorie amount.

Basal Metabolic Rate (BMR)

To determine the amount of calories we should consume daily, we start with something called our basal metabolic rate (BMR). This is the amount of calories we need to consume to maintain our normal bodily functions. Your BMR can be calculated using the Harris-Benedict Formula for women:

$$BMR = 655 + (4.35 \text{ x weight in pounds}) + (4.7 \text{ x height in inches}) - (4.7 \text{ x age in years})$$

Again, unless you are a super mathematician, or you just enjoy solving complicated formulas like this, please consider using one of the many easy online BMR calculators like bmrcalculator.org. All you need to input is your age, height, weight, and gender, and it does the calculation for you.

Building on our example above, using this formula, let's calculate Tracy Triathlete's BMR:

$$\text{Tracy Triathlete is 145 lbs., 5' 5", and 40 years old.}$$
$$BMR = 655 + (4.35 \text{ x } 145) + (4.7 \text{ x } 65) - (4.7 \text{ x } 40)$$
$$BMR = 1,403 \text{ calories}$$

This is the approximate number of calories Tracy needs daily to maintain her current weight without consideration for exercise.

However, for athletes like yourself, you may have to increase this amount based on the number of days per week you are exercising and at what intensity. Here is a simple formula you can use to determine how much you need to increase your BMR to adjust for your daily exercise and intensity.

Multiply your BMR by the appropriate activity factor as follows:

Activity Factor

Sedentary (little or no exercise): BMR x 1.2

Lightly active (light exercise/sports 1 to 3 days/week): BMR x 1.375

Moderately active (moderate exercise/sports 3 to 5 days/week): BMR x 1.55

Very active (hard exercise/sports 6 to 7 days a week): BMR x 1.725

Extra active (very hard exercise/sports and physical job or twice a day training): BMR x 1.9

Your final number is the approximate number of calories you need each day to maintain your weight.

On average, Tracy Triathlete moderately exercises five days a week. In order for her to maintain her weight, she should consume approximately 2,175 calories per day calculated as follows:

$$\text{BMR} = 1{,}403 \text{ (as per the Harris-Benedict Formula)}$$
$$\text{x } 1.55 \text{ (activity factor)} = 2{,}175 \text{ calories per day}$$

As we mentioned earlier though, most women are in a position where they want to lose a few pounds before the triathlon season begins. And for those few women who want to gain a few pounds, you can use these approaches as well.

We start by determining the number of calories we need to consume to lose 1 pound of body weight a week. Anything more than 1 to 1.5 pounds per week is pretty unrealistic and is not usually an effective approach in keeping that weight off. Let's start with one of the basic calorie-reduction methods.

The "500-Calorie Reduction Per Day" Approach

A very popular weight-management method that athletes have used to either increase or decrease their body weight is the "500-calorie reduction per day" approach. It is based on the fact that 1 pound is the equivalent of 3,500 calories, which, divided by seven days in a week, equals 500 calories per day. If an athlete increases her net calorie intake by about 500 calories a day over her BMR, she will typically gain about a pound per week. Likewise, if she decreases her average net calorie intake by an average of about 500 calories a day, she will typically lose about a pound per week.

Let's again use Tracy Triathlete as our example. She would like to drop her weight from 145 pounds to 140 pounds with about two months to go before her racing season begins.

Example: Tracy Triathlete: BMR + activity factor = 2,175 calories per day (as calculated above) – 500 calories per day = 1,675 net daily calories

Using the "500-calorie reduction per day" formula, Tracy would have to consume about 1,675 calories per day to lose approximately 1 pound per week.

Although this is a good approach for a lot of average-size women, for a larger woman or a smaller woman, the 500-calorie rule may be too small or too large a percentage of their current body weight. For these women, we suggest another approach for your consideration.

The "11 Calories Per Body Pound" Approach

This is a calculation based on the estimation that to maintain our current weight and cover our daily activities, we need to consume about 14 calories per pound of body weight per day, and to lose weight at a healthy rate, we should consume about 11 calories per pound of body weight per day.

Many nutritional experts suggest a reasonable daily target of 10 calories per pound of body weight for most people trying to lose weight. But that figure applies to heavier, if not obese, sedentary people. Through our work with female endurance athletes who are just looking to sculpt their bodies down to race weight, we find that a daily target of 11 calories per pound of body weight is usually optimal.

Here is an example of the "11 calories per body pound" approach as applied to Tracy Triathlete:

Tracy Triathlete: Female, 145 lbs., 5' 5", 40 years old
145 lbs. x 11 calories per body pound = 1,595 daily calories

If we compare the two approaches and the results of each test based on our example of Tracy Triathlete, the difference is about 80 calories per day as outlined below. This is very comparable and gives you the option to go with the higher or lower number based on your experience in losing weight.

Comparison of "500-calorie reduction per day" approach and "11 calories per body pound" approach for Tracy Triathlete:

500-calorie reduction: 1,675 (as calculated above)
11 calories per body pound: 1,595 (as calculated above)
Difference = 80 calories per day

For Tracy Triathlete to lose weight at a healthy rate, she should target a consumption of approximately 1,595 to 1,675 calories per day.

Tracking Your Calories and Exercise

Now for the hard part: actually following through and working every day to eat the proper amount of calories to get you to your ideal weight.

Working with many athletes for many years, we have found that the easiest way is to track your food and drink every day using an online application or mobile phone application like myfitnesspal.com or loseit.com. These are two great online applications that help keep you in check every day and make sure you are ending on or about your desired calories, even considering your exercise, as you will record that as well. This is no easy task, and results can be slow depending on your age and overall genetics. So be patient, be consistent, and you will eventually get to your ideal weight.

Fueling and Hydration for Training and Racing

Now that we have talked about our daily nutrition, let's take a look at how to most effectively fuel and hydrate during training and racing. Here are five truisms you should know about fueling and hydration:

1. There are no magic bullets to fueling and hydration for training and racing other than experimenting, testing, and retesting in training.
2. You have to learn to maximize your healthy level of calorie and fluid intake during training and racing. For most athletes this

means replacing close to 100 percent of their fluids and 33 to 50 percent of their calories lost. It is a process to determine what is optimal for you, and that doesn't happen in one training session.

3. Our fueling and hydration needs are unique to us. What works for someone else may not work for you.

4. Keep it simple. The simpler your fueling and hydration plan, the more likely you will be able to execute your plan. This starts with knowing what will be offered on the race course and practicing with it in training.

5. Stick with your fueling and hydration plan—don't be distracted by the excitement of the race or other diversions. Stick with your plan.

In our decades of training and racing, we have heard it all, from "I just couldn't stomach the energy drink they had on the course" to "I threw up in the swim" to "I just couldn't take in another sugary drink!" This is why it is so important to repeatedly practice your exact fueling and hydration plan each week in training. We need to make it second nature and stick with it to perfection on race day.

An IronFit Moment

Carbo-Loading

It seems women have a harder time than most men carbo-loading even the day before a race, let alone two days before. This is not scientific but anecdotal from our many years of experience coaching women athletes. And it makes sense, since often women just can't eat as much as men. However, this is not necessarily a bad thing. Studies have shown that women appear to burn more fat and less carbohydrate than men during endurance exercise. So carbo-loading may not be so much of a factor for women. Since ordinarily most women have more fat than men, this is a good thing. What this means is that for events lasting two or more hours, women will outlast their male counterparts in terms of expending their supply of liver and muscle glycogen, hence they don't need to do as much carbo-loading. The studies don't conclude why women have a greater reliance on fat than men, but it has been thought to relate to the effects of estrogen on metabolism. Also, it is thought that estrogen may protect muscles from exercise-induced damage under some circumstances. This is supported by actual performances of men and women in ultradistance races. The longer the race, the more likely it is that women outperform men.

Determining Your Own Hydration Needs

The easiest way to determine your hydration needs is through proper testing in training. We have developed the simple, basic Sweat Rate Test protocol, which we have successfully used over the years with the athletes we coach. This can be done for swimming, cycling, and running and in varying temperatures, heart rates, or perceived effort.

Our Sweat Rate Test protocol is as follows:

1. Weigh yourself (without clothing) prior to your cardio activity (swim, bike, or run).

2. Perform your activity for at least 60 minutes at a heart rate equal to 75 percent of your maximum heart rate (MHR).

3. During the 60 minutes of activity, very evenly consume 16 ounces of water.

4. Weigh yourself (without clothing) immediately after your 60-minute activity has been completed.

5. Complete the following calculations:
   a. Weight before − weight after = net weight loss
   b. Net weight loss + 1.0 pound (16 oz. of water consumed) = hourly sweat loss

(Note: 1 pound = 16 ounces)

To get a better understanding of the Sweat Rate Test, let's use Tracy Triathlete to demonstrate. She is going to ride her bike indoors on a trainer for 60 minutes at about 75 percent of her maximum heart rate and the temperature inside is about 70°F. She weighed herself before the activity and was 145 pounds and then again after the 60-minute test and she weighed 144 pounds. During the 60 minutes she consumes 16 ounces of water. Using that information, the following is the calculation to determine her Sweat Rate:

Weight before = 145.0 pounds

Weight after = 144.0 pounds

Difference =   1.0 pound

Weight loss: 145.0 – 144.0 = 1.0 pound (or 16 ounces)

Hourly Sweat Rate: 1.0 pound (16 oz.) + 1.0 pound (16 oz. of water consumed) = 2.0 pounds (32 oz.)

Tracy lost 16 ounces, despite replenishing with 16 ounces of fluid. Therefore, she is down a total of 32 ounces for the hour. This indicates that under similar conditions (i.e., temperature, heart rate level, and activity), she should replenish fluids at a rate of about 32 ounces per hour.

This is a great starting point, and it gives you an idea of what your hydration needs are and how to plan hydration replacement for training sessions and racing.

But as we all know, conditions on race day can be different, so what do we do? If we are planning to race in a warmer climate than 70°F, then we should retest again at the expected climate on race day. Maybe that is 80°F, so Tracy Triathlete should perform the test again at that temperature and see what the test yields.

Let's say she does that test and she loses 1.5 pounds, resulting in 40 ounces lost. This would indicate that on race day, she would need to take in a range of about 32 to 40 ounces of fluids if the expected temperature is between 70°F and 80°F.

Training and Racing Hydration

Based on the results of your Sweat Rate Test(s), you can determine how much hydration you require hourly and start practicing with that amount of hydration in training. You should train with the energy drink that will be available to you on the race course unless you plan to carry all of your own hydration sources with you.

You want to determine your required race hydration (i.e., ounces per hour) to support racing at various temperatures, event durations, and intensity. Practice what you plan to do during the race in training. If you expect it to be much warmer during the race, you need to consider taking in more hydration. If it's a bit cooler, you may not have to take in quite as much. And you will be able to determine this by performing the Sweat Rate Test described above in varying temperatures and intensities.

In previous books we have highlighted the following racing hydration data for a sampling of eight athletes in our more elite-level age groups:

Fluid ounces consumed per hour: 24 to 43 oz. (range)

Fluid ounces (oz.) to body weight (lbs.) ratio: 0.20 (average); 0.15 to 0.24 (range)

Our eight athletes consumed on average 33.5 ounces of fluid per hour while racing, and the range among the eight athletes varied from a low of 24 ounces to a high of 43 ounces. Since size and body mass account for some of this difference, we also looked at this data on the basis of ounces of fluid per pound of body weight. The average ratio for the group was 0.20 ounces of fluid per pound of body weight, with a range of 0.15 to 0.24 ounces per pound of body weight.

This information is valuable when determining your optimal race hydration strategy and especially your hourly hydration needs. In addition to performing the Sweat Rate Test and testing the results in training, we suggest you also check your results against this sampling of eight experienced athletes on the basis of fluid ounces per hour to body weight.

By simply using the above Sweat Rate Test protocol, comparing the results with the results of this eight-athlete sampling, and then testing and fine-tuning the results in training, you will determine your optimal race hydration replacement plan.

Once we know how much we want to take in and how often, then, logistically, we need to determine how we will get that hydration in during the race. Most likely you will start with two to four bottles on your bike depending on the race distance, then you'll possibly take bottles from the aid stations along the course. Or like some of our athletes doing longer-distance races, you may want to consider using a CamelBak to ensure you get your fluids in timely and evenly throughout your race.

On the run, it's the same thing: You can either take your hydration from the aid stations or carry a fuel belt, handheld bottle, or even a CamelBak for really long events.

But whatever you decide, plan for it and practice that plan.

Pre-Race Hydration

On the morning of a race, we suggest you start your hydration as soon as you wake up, which should be about three hours before the event, and you should continue to gradually hydrate right up to the start of the race. You should practice this as part of your pre-training routine as well.

How much fluid should you consume in the morning prior to a race? A good place to start is to consider what successful athletes are doing and then to do your own testing in training. In previous books we have highlighted the following pre-racing hydration data for a sampling of eight athletes in our more elite-level age groups:

Pre-Race Hydration Data

- Average fluid oz. consumed: 58.5 (ranging from 45 to 72 oz.)
- Average fluid (oz.) to body weight (lbs.) ratio: 0.36 (ranging from 0.28 to 0.43)

The same eight elite coached athletes referred to earlier in this chapter have an average of 58.5 ounces of fluids within the three hours leading up to their races, with a range of 45 ounces to 72 ounces. To help adjust for differences in athlete size and body mass, we also consider pre-race hydration on the basis of average fluid per pound of body weight, which is 0.36 ounces per pound of body weight, with a range of 0.28 to 0.43 ounces.

This is valuable information as you determine your optimal pre-race hydration amounts. We suggest you use these ranges as a starting point and then fine-tune your specific amounts through frequent testing in training. Practice this in training so you are well prepared to do it before your big race.

Tip: Utilize mostly energy drinks and limit your water intake to about 8 ounces of your total hydration amounts to avoid any sodium dilution and potential hyponatremia.

Training and Race Fueling

You can fuel with solids and/or liquids. Athletes who experience gastro issues during training and racing may decide to take in only fluid calories. For most athletes, though, you want to consider fueling calorie sources like energy gels, Chomps, Bloks, or even energy bars. In our experience most athletes consume about 93 to 100 percent carbohydrates during the race and only about 0 to 7 percent protein and fat. So again, use this as a guide to determine the sources you will fuel with.

How much calorie replacement do we need? We find that most athletes should evenly replace between one-third and one-half of their calories utilized during the race. The longer it takes the athlete to complete the race, the closer we should typically be to targeting a 50 percent calorie replenishment.

So, for example, if the activity burns calories at a rate of 900 per hour, then you should be replacing your calories at a rate of 300 to 450 calories per hour (i.e., one-third of 900 equals 300 and one-half of 900 equals 450). You should consider using this estimated range during training.

The easiest way to determine what will work best for you in a race is to test it in training. We like to recommend, when possible, to keep it simple. Practice with the fueling in training that you will use or will be available to you during your race both on the bike and run portions of the race, if any.

From our experience in coaching athletes for many years and from our own experiences, we have developed ranges of calories and a ratio of calories to body weight consumed during racing that you can experiment with yourself in training and then ultimately use for racing. In previous books we have highlighted the following race fueling data for a sampling of eight athletes of our more elite-level age groups:

Race Fueling Data:

- Average calories per hour: 404 (ranging from 270 to 537)
- Average calories per hour per body weight (lbs.): 2.6 (ranging from 1.7 to 3.3)

The average calorie intake for these eight elite-level athletes was about 404 calories per hour, and the athletes ranged from 270 to 537 calories per hour. Obviously, the bigger athletes typically had the higher totals and the smaller athletes the lower totals. So to get a better apples-to-apples comparison, we have included the second statistic, which indicates that on average these athletes consumed 2.6 calories for every pound of body weight.

For example, an athlete who weighed 155 pounds consumed about 400 calories per hour (i.e., 155 x 2.6 = 403). This is very helpful information as you determine your optimal amount of calories per hour in your fueling plan.

Our suggestion is to use the two above criteria (ratio of calorie intake to calories utilized and ratio of calorie intake to body weight) to help determine the optimal calories for racing. Once you determine your calorie amount, test it frequently in all of your longer training sessions to see how it makes you feel. Then adjust and fine-tune as you train to arrive at the optimal amount for you.

The next question is, logistically, how will you access those calories during the race? Will you use a fuel belt during the run to carry your energy gels in a flask or in your pocket in separate packages, or do you plan to get them at specific aid stations along the course? How many bike bottles will you carry on your bike and how many will you take from the aid stations, if any? These are the questions you will have answered well before the race by knowing what is or is not being offered on the course.

Another important point to make is that you want to take in your hydration and fueling evenly throughout every training and racing hour. We suggest taking in hydration at least every 10–15 minutes and fueling every 30 to 40 minutes.

Pre-Race Fueling

Your pre-race fueling will differ based on the duration and intensity of your race. It should consist primarily of carbohydrates about 70 to 80 percent with some fat and protein about 20 to 30 percent. The amount of calories will differ based on the individual and the anticipated intensity and duration of the event.

From our experience of coaching athletes for many years and our own experiences, we have developed ranges of calories and a ratio of calories to body weight consumed during training that you can experiment with yourself in training too and then ultimately use for racing. In previous books we have highlighted the following pre-race fueling data for a sampling of eight athletes in our more elite-level age groups:

Pre-Race Fueling Data:

- Average calories consumed: 951 (ranging from 690 to 1,212)
- Average calories to body weight (lbs.) ratio: 6.6 (ranging from 5.7 to 7.3)

The same eight elite coached athletes consume an average of about 951 calories in the three hours before their races, with a range of from 690 to 1,212. To help adjust for differences in athlete size and body mass, we also consider pre-race calories on the basis of average calories per pound of body weight, which is 6.6 calories per pound, with a range of 5.7 to 7.3.

This is also valuable information as you determine your optimal pre-race fueling amounts.

For most any distance race, you will want to finish fueling with solids at least one to two hours before the race to be sure your food is digested and your stomach is settled. However, you can continue with liquid fueling sources right up until race time.

There is no substitute for practicing in training with what you plan to fuel and hydrate with and when during your race. We cannot emphasize enough that you must practice in training or it will not happen on race day. The reality is that when race day comes it should be a slam-dunk!

Following is the third of seven motivating profiles of an inspiring female triathlete.

ATHLETE SUCCESS STORY:
MELISSA SILVERMAN

Melissa Silverman has a busy lifestyle. Melissa has been married for over thirty years, has three adult children and one grandson, and works with her husband in their family ophthalmic practice. Amazingly, she has also been training for and racing in triathlons for the past eight years.

Melissa is also a cancer survivor. While going through radiation treatments back in 2005, she received a pamphlet from the Leukemia Society's Team in Training program urging her to participate in one of their events. It seemed like just the right thing at the right time, and she and her husband Cary signed up for their Tour de Tucson 109-mile cycling event. After successfully finishing this daunting ride and feeling like she wanted another challenge, she signed up for her first triathlon. And as they say, the rest is history.

Melissa enjoys sprint and standard distances the most and competes in several each year. She finds the training time commitment for these distances to be more manageable and it allows for a more balanced lifestyle . . . especially in terms of family and friends.

Melissa doesn't consider her greatest achievement in triathlon to be any one single racing performance, but more how she has grown as a person through triathlon. She has become stronger through the many emotional ups and downs of training and racing. She has faced injuries along the way and mechanical breakdowns during races, but she has always found the strength to carry on to the finish and overcome each and every challenge along the way. Her mental toughness has grown, and challenges that may have thrown her for a loop years ago are taken in stride today. Most important, she has learned a lot about herself through the process and she is very proud of who she has discovered herself to be.

Melissa's advice for other women athletes: "Have a sense of self. Know who you are. Work hard. Give it all you can. Don't give up at the first upset. There is something to learn from every single race you do. And remember: You are good enough! Be proud of yourself for taking on this challenge."

CHAPTER 4

Race Selection and Goal Setting for Women

Commitment leads to action.
Action brings your dream closer.

—*Marcia Wieder, author and speaker*
on health issues

n this chapter we provide guidance on how to select the optimal races for you and also how to set the most effective goals. Once you have determined the best races and goals for you, we will share our secrets on how to make your goals even more powerful in driving your success.

Race Selection Challenges for Women

There are so many factors to consider, so while selecting the best races is challenging enough for triathletes in general, it is even more so for women. In addition to all of the usual factors, women need to also decide between open races with men or women-only races. Then there are many other considerations including race distance, travel time, topography, and your strengths and weakness.

Women-Only Races and Swim Waves

While much of the criteria for selecting your race distance are pretty much the same for everyone, women have a whole other layer of complication they need to consider. Do you want to race with men, race women-only races, or perhaps race with men but only in races with separate women-only swim waves?

If it's your first triathlon, you may very well want to consider one of the women-only race series. They are usually at the sprint distance and they mostly go out of their way to make their races inviting and nonthreatening to newcomers. They often provide "swim angels" to assist first-timers in the swim. We coach many elite athletes today who have told us that they would never had even tried triathlon in the first place had it not been for women-only races. The thought of an open-water swim start with testosterone-charged twentysomething men was not their idea of fun. Yet, many years and races later, these same women are totally comfortable racing with men.

Beth Poore, one of our coached athletes, can count among her many athletic accomplishments over the past four years that of being a four-time Iron-Distance Triathlon finisher. What's more, she has lowered her times in each

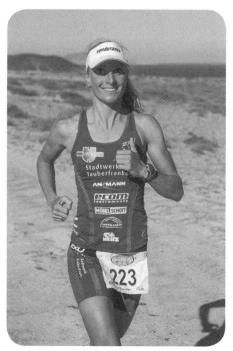

Pro triathlete and Ironman champion Heidi Sessner / *James Mitchell Photography*

successive race. It's hard to believe that someone so accomplished would ever have had doubts about even trying a sprint triathlon in the first place, but Beth says that she would never have even tried a triathlon had she not seen the advertisement for a women-only sprint triathlon. The advertisement was for the Danskin Triathlon Series, which, as we mentioned earlier, may be responsible for bringing tens of thousands of women into our sport. Beth said that the advertisement made the women-only triathlon seem so inviting, nonthreatening, and supportive, that she felt compelled to give it a try. And as they say, the rest is history.

But unlike Beth, who moved on to open races with men, some women start with the women-only races and never leave. They enjoy them and prefer them, so why leave?

Now that the sport has grown so much, even when the race is not a women-only race, the swim waves are usually women-only. This is a big plus because although you will be racing with men eventually in the race, at least at the very start of the race, you will only be swimming with women. This is extremely helpful because this is the most crowded part of the race and athlete-to-athlete contact is most likely.

So, check the websites of the races you are considering to see exactly how they are set up. As we said, most races now have women-only swim waves, although the Ironman races organized by the World Triathlon Corporation are all, or mostly all, mass swim starts with both men and women. But race formats continue to change and evolve as the sport grows.

We suggest you always check in advance to see what the situation will be before signing up. If it's your first race, however, we suggest you consider a women-only race.

An IronFit Moment

Tips for Swimming with Men

Some of our coached female athletes are extremely strong swimmers, and the men racing with them will be wise to keep an eye out for them, rather than the other way around. But for female athletes who are not strong swimmers, the start of the race can be intimidating, if not dangerous. For example, if you are a fifty-year-old first-timer, you definitely want to position yourself wisely at the start and avoid having some crazy testosterone-charged twentysomething male competitor rudely decide to swim over, rather than around, you. It's a shame that this type of thing can happen in our sport, but the important thing to know is that it can easily be avoided with proper planning. To help make your racing experience the best it can be, please consider the following tips for swim starts . . . especially swim starts with men:

- Position yourself at the start conservatively back from the front. Don't line up in front unless you are a very strong swimmer. If you don't belong there, it will surely be a race-spoiling experience. If you are an average swimmer, position yourself halfway back. As you become a faster swimmer and a more experienced triathlete over time, move up accordingly. If you are a weak swimmer or a beginner, start at the back of the pack and avoid contact completely. In fact, if you are an absolute beginner, please consider waiting 30 to 60 seconds after the starting gun fires. Take a couple of long relaxed breaths, and then begin to swim at an easy and relaxed pace. You are not planning to win the race, so those 30 to 60 seconds will be meaningless. But you sure will have a much more relaxed, fun, and stress-free swim.

- Now that you know how far back from the front line you should position yourself, should you go to the left, the right, or perhaps the middle? If you are a beginner, the middle is definitely a no-no. It's the most stressful and dangerous place to swim because you will be boxed in from all sides and likely to encounter a great deal of physical contact. Instead, position yourself to the side of the pack that is your nonbreathing side. In other words, if you breathe to the left, line up on the far right of the pack. This means that there will be no swimmers behind you on your blind side and you will be able to see the swimmers to your left when you breathe. This will help to avoid collisions.

- Now that you know exactly where to position yourself at the start, the next key element to focus on is to swim straight. When the gun goes off, make sure you are swimming in a straight line. (If you are not sure you can do this, see the drills designed to help you to do so in Chapter 14.) Very often an athlete thinks that other swimmers keep swimming into them, but it's actually they who are swimming into the other swimmers. By learning to swim in a straight line, you will reduce the amount of contact you have with the other swimmers and you will have a faster and more efficient swim.

Race Distance

Now that you have decided between women-only races and open races with men, the next consideration is race distance. The two key factors here are your experience level and what motivates you. Our suggestion is to start small and then gradually build from there. So, if your next triathlon will be your first triathlon, we suggest making it a Sprint Distance Triathlon. Then, once you successfully accomplish your Sprint Distance Triathlon, feel free to move up to the next triathlon distance. So after starting with a Sprint, if you think you would like to race a Standard Distance, go for it. Likewise, after a successful Standard Distance triathlon, you may want to take on a Half Iron-Distance. And finally, after your Half Iron-Distance Triathlon, you may decide to take on the full Iron-Distance.

But please do not feel you need to move up to the longer distances if you do not really want to. We coach plenty of athletes who enjoy the short course races the most and that is what they focus on. One of the issues we see in the sport is that there is a lot of hype around the longer distances and athletes often feel obligated and pressured to move up to them. Some athletes even start out in the sport with their very first race being at the Iron-Distance, which we really do not recommend.

For long-term success and enjoyment of the sport, find the distances that you enjoy the most and don't be steered away by what someone else says you "have to do." Ignore the noise. Every racing distance is a worthy one. Find the distance that best fits your lifestyle. Then, enjoy the challenge and enjoy the journey.

If you do decide you want to race long course, then we suggest you gradually build up to it one distance at a time and play it safe.

Other Race Selection Criteria

After you have decided on the race distance and women-only versus open races with men, there are several other factors we suggest you consider.

Not only will the optimal type of triathlon vary from athlete to athlete, there is also a different set of criteria for an athlete's first and subsequent triathlons. Many additional factors come into play: the athlete's individual strengths and weaknesses versus the topography of the race, timing considerations, climate, and many more. For example, while a professional woman may have work schedule issues to coordinate her races with, a stay-at-home mom may have her kids' school and vacation schedules to deal with, and a mom with a career outside the home may have both.

Following are the additional factors we suggest you consider in selecting your races:

- **Strength and weaknesses:** Consider if you want to select a race that favors your strengths as an athlete. If one of your primary goals is to improve your placing within your age group, it will be helpful to select a course that suits you well and gives you more of an advantage over your competitors. For example, if you are a strong swimmer, you may want to select a race that has a non-wet-suit swim and/or a swim course that is choppy or has a strong current.

- **Topography:** Do you prefer a very hilly course or a very flat course? If it's all about improving your placing in your age group, then this relates to the "strengths and weaknesses" described above and you will want to match the topography of the course to your strengths. But if your goal is time-related, it may make more sense for you to select a course that is flat and fast. These are just two possibilities. We know many athletes who are not that interested in their time or their placing and instead select courses with attractive topography just because they enjoy the views out on the course and, of course, the personal challenge.

- **Climate:** Consider whether or not you can be prepared for the likely weather and climate on race day before signing up for a particular race. If you are living in an area that is cold and racing at a location that will be hot and humid, it will likely have a negative impact on your performance. It takes our bodies several days to adjust to a different climate, and the more different, the more days it will take. A common example of this is the Hawaii Ironman in October. Many of the athletes we coach who are training in North America and northern Europe are not immediately prepared for the heat and humidity of Hawaii. An athlete needs to select her races with this in mind and be ready to either travel to the race location very early to acclimate or use heat acclimation techniques in their training.

- **Altitude:** Do you live and train at sea level? If so, it may not be wise to select a race located at a high altitude. While arriving early can help you adjust to higher altitude, you may be giving up a big advantage to your competitors. In general, we suggest that if you live and train at low altitude that you primarily race at low altitude.

- **Timing considerations:** As briefly touched on above, it's easy to determine how long you need to prepare for your races based on the training programs in this book. We suggest you use this information to help select your races. Select your races so they best fit the training plans in this book as well as your own personal schedule (e.g., vacation time, work schedule, family schedule, etc.).

- **Travel considerations:** Consider all travel issues before selecting your race. There are thousands of wonderful races all across the world. Depending on your location, you can probably select a race that's so close by that you can sleep in your own bed and drive there the morning of the race. Or you can fly many time zones away to a race on the other side of the planet . . . and everything in between. Either option is fine—just do your homework in advance and know what to expect. While traveling can be fun and exciting, it can also add a lot of complications to your racing experience. This may be fine if you are an experienced veteran, but if you are a newbie, it may be better to try to keep your traveling as simple as possible and to a minimum.

- **Cost considerations:** This relates somewhat to "Travel Considerations" above. The travel expense of driving to a race on race morning may cost you a quarter tank of gasoline. On the other hand, the travel to that race on the other side of the planet may cost you thousands of dollars in the form of airfare, hotels, local transportation, meals, etc. The other big cost consideration is race fees. These vary widely. One of our coached athletes registered recently for the New York Triathlon Club's Central Park Duathlon in April to use as an early season tune-up for an Iron-Distance in Lake Placid, New York, about four months later. The race fee for the former was $70 and for the latter was $700—ten times more expensive! These are obviously very different types of great race experiences, but they serve as a good example of how much entry fees can vary from one race to another.

Setting Empowering Goals

While having exciting races on your calendar will definitely motivate you in your triathlon journey, by properly marrying your races with highly effective goals, you will take your motivation to an even higher level.

Proper goal setting includes setting "primary" goals and "stretch" goals, as well as short- and long-term goals. We will explain each in the following sections. We will also discuss the pros and cons of "qualitative" goals versus "quantitative" goals.

Primary Goals

We define a "primary goal" as the minimum goal in your mind that will constitute success. In the broadest sense, we feel that virtually every race is a success. Even when things go terribly wrong, there are always many lessons that can be learned and valuable information to be taken away. But what we are talking about with a primary goal is one that, prior to the race, you would consider to be the minimum level of positive outcomes.

For a first-time triathlete, a good primary goal may be to simply finish the race in good health and good spirits. For an experienced athlete a good primary goal might be to set a new personal best time at a particular race distance. These are both good primary goals because while they are not easily achievable, they are definitely achievable if you really do your best to prepare and race well. These goals will help us to do exactly that.

Stretch Goals

We define stretch goals as goals that are possible, but in fact so challenging that they are not *probable*. Almost everything has to work out perfectly for us to achieve them. Perhaps they don't require a miracle, but the stars definitely need to fall into alignment.

A good example of a stretch goal might be to win your age group when you have never done so before. Maybe you have come in somewhere in the top ten before but have not really come close to winning. Sure, it's not likely that you will win your age group in your next race, but you have "been in the neighborhood before," and now that you are working with a new training plan, you think you have a shot at it.

Short-Term versus Long-Term Goals

We consider short-term goals to be goals for the next twelve months and long-term goals to be goals for beyond the current year. An example of a good short-term goal might be to complete your first Half Iron-Distance Triathlon this year and a good long-term goal might be to complete a full Iron-Distance Triathlon within the next three years. For the best motivation and results, we suggest you consider having both short- and long-term goals.

Having worked with hundreds of athletes over the years, it has been our experience that short-term goals have the immediacy of helping you to be motivated to get out and train today. Knowing that the "day of truth" is coming soon allows us to break through procrastination and feel the urgency of near-term.

It has been our experience that long-term goals put everything into prospective and keep us heading in the right direction. While short-term goals help us to "get out the door" and swim, bike, and run, long-term goals encourage us to make and maintain truely positive lifestyle changes.

Qualitative versus Quantitative Goals

While we typically encourage our coached athletes to set quantitative goals versus qualitative goals, we realize that this is not best for all athletes, especially for women. While we have coached many women who prefer and do best with very specific quantitative goals, we also see a lot of female athletes who prefer softer, more qualitative goals.

An example of a quantitative goal is the goal to race under 2.5 hours for the Standard Distance Triathlon. It's quantitative in the sense that you either do it or you don't do it. Your time is either under 2.5 hours or it's not. There is nothing subjective about it.

An example of a qualitative goal is the aspiration to "feel good about my race." This athlete is not really that motivated by her race times. She wants it to be a fun and enjoyable experience. If she finishes the race and feels good about it, it means she is likely to want to race more. And that defines success for her. So this is a good type of goal for her. Another common quantitative goal for some women after having children or not having exercised regularly since college is to get back into a consistent training routine and back to a healthy lifestyle. And putting a triathlon goal on the calendar may be just the thing they need.

We suggest you consider what motivates you the most—qualitative or quantitative goals—or perhaps a mix of both, and then plan your goals accordingly.

An IronFit Moment

Following are the six current goals for experienced triathlete Tracy Triathlete as they appear at the top of her training schedule. As you will see, Tracy sets goals in all of the categories we have discussed: primary, stretch, short-term, long-term, qualitative, and quantitative.

2016 Goals:

Short-Term: 1) Set a new personal best time @ the Standard Distance Triathlon (primary goal); 2) Qualify for the first time for the Standard Distance National Championships (stretch goal); 3) Develop a more positive self-image through triathlon (qualitative goal); **Long Term:** 4) Complete an Iron-Distance Triathlon within the next three years (primary goal); 5) Qualify for the Hawaii Ironman World Championships within the next five years (stretch goal); 6) Positively impact my friends, family, and coworkers through my athletics (qualitative goal).

Supercharge Your Goals by "Posting" Them

Probably the single most successful technique for supercharging our goals is to "post" them. We start by listing our coached athletes' goals prominently at the very top of their training schedules so they see them every day. We also encourage them to take the power of goals to another level by posting them at locations in their home and/or place of work to be reminded of them frequently. Or use whatever social media (Facebook, Twitter, etc.) motivates you and provides you support from your family and friends.

What we are talking about here is actually creating old-school handwritten little signs or posting them on your Facebook page with your goals written on them. A simple example of one might be as follows:

Columbia Triathlon
Standard Distance PR
Top 3 AG
Healthy and in good spirits

This athlete plans to race in one of our favorite Standard Distance races, the Columbia Triathlon in Ellicott City, Maryland, and has the primary goal of finishing in a new personal best time, the stretch goal of placing in the top three in her age group, and the qualitative goal of finishing the race "healthy and in good spirits."

Posting goals works great with primary goals, stretch goals, qualitative goals, or all three, as in the above example. Just go with whatever you find motivates you the most.

One of the most productive places to post goals is on your bathroom mirror, as that is the first thing many athletes see each day. Other popular places include your work area or your workout area, or keep it as your screensaver on your smartphone or computer.

There is a wonderfully motivating power to posting goals. It keeps us focused on what we want to achieve and it helps us to make wise decisions each and every day that will positively impact our ability to achieve our goals.

What if Your True Goal Is to "Beat My Training Buddy"?

It's funny, but many times when we ask one of our coached athletes what her goal is, she tells us it's to "beat my friend" or to "beat my training buddy." While we appreciate the honesty . . . and we get it . . . we have found that this type of goal is not a particularly positive or good one.

The most effective goals are ones that are positive and uplifting with the context of healthy competition, while the concept of "beating" someone comes from a somewhat negative place. Goals that mark improvement in our fitness and performance are much more positive and motivating. After all, if you don't improve, but you still manage to finish ahead of your friend, not much has really been accomplished. Our suggestion is to take the highest road and set goals that are positive and uplifting and more self-focused.

In fact, if you are going to make goals that involve your friends, bring them into the loop. We know several groups of female triathletes who have fun goals like traveling together to at least three races per year. What a great way to build camaraderie and create fun experiences with your training buddies! But be aware that while friendly competition can be a good thing, it can also distract you from your ultimate goal or goals.

This chapter presents the fourth of seven motivating profiles of an inspiring female triathlete.

ATHLETE SUCCESS STORY:
MARCIA POSTALLIAN

Marcia Postallian is an Adult Nurse Practitioner in the Veterans Administration specializing in primary care, and she's an experienced triathlete of over eighteen years and forty races. Marcia enjoys the faster short-course races the most and recently had the honor of representing her country as part of Team USA at the Triathlon World Championships in London.

It all started for Marcia at a sprint distance event in Michigan back in 1996. She was encouraged by a fellow swimmer in her Masters Swim program. Her friend warned her, though, that if she wanted to be competitive, she would need to upgrade from her mountain bike. *Competitive?* Marcia thought. All she hoped for at the time was to make it safely back to shore on the swim leg. But that was a long time ago, and now she competes at the very highest levels. Marcia loved her first triathlon experience and continues to enjoy the supportive and collaborative triathlon environment today.

Sure, there have been setbacks along the way—injuries and other of life's little hurdles. But Marcia has persevered and taken them all in stride. Marcia says that she receives strength from the veterans she cares for who bravely carry on through a lot more than a simple athletic injury.

As many endurance athletes have told us over the years, Marcia says that she receives a great therapeutic benefit from her training. It has helped her through the ups and downs of life. In fact, Marcia credits her swimming, cycling, and running as key to helping her through the sad time of her divorce and putting her right back on track for happier times.

As an experienced and accomplished athlete, Marcia is often asked for her advice on how best to get started. Marcia encourages them to join Masters Swimming, a triathlon club, or a running club. "There you will find many likeminded people who will help you on your way," Marcia says, adding that, "If you find it difficult to break the ice, ask them what sports nutrition they use, what kind of bike they ride, or what kind of sports bra chafes less, and they'll respond with great enthusiasm." Marcia also suggests that newbies start with a Just-Finish training program for their first race and/or hire a coach if you have the resources. Finally, Marcia says, "Women are stronger than they think, and training and racing are one way to see this strength in ourselves."

CHAPTER 5

Triathlon Equipment for the Female Triathlete

Men are from Mars, women are from Venus.

—John Gray, PhD, relationship counselor and author

The biggest difference we find between women and men triathletes is a desire for the latest and greatest gadgets. Most men want to have the fanciest Garmin watch and latest great high-tech bike, and most women just want a bike that works and that they don't have to mess around with. It is almost comical when you compare the majority of men to women in this area of the sport.

In our experience, it is not to say that women are not interested in having a great bike or having a fancy heart rate monitor, but it is not a priority for most women. If they can get on their bikes and ride without any issues and can use their heart rate monitors without a problem, they are happy.

However, as much as we are not "gadget coaches" either, there are definitely some basic things you should know about your equipment, from safety reasons to just common sense.

We'll break this down into the three disciplines of the sport—swimming, cycling, and running—and, finally, the triathlon gear.

Swimming Equipment

More often than not, most women will figure out which swimsuit, cap, and goggles fit them best just by going to their local swim shop and trying on a suit, cap, and several pairs of goggles. To test the goggles to see if they fit, press them to your face and see if they hold without use of the strap. If they fall off immediately, they probably are not the correct ones for you. There are also goggles that are a little bit larger for open-water swimming, but try them first to make sure you like them. From our experience, a lot of women like them because they don't make marks around your eyes, but in the pool they can lead to too much head rotation when breathing.

Another gadget you might use in swimming is a pull buoy, which is a floating device that you hold between your thighs at crotch height. It can help to develop some upper body strength and also simulates wearing a wet suit by holding up your legs. Your Masters Swim coach may have you use it during a practice, and our swim workouts have "pull" sets also. We'll talk more about swim technique in Chapter 14, but you can also use the pull buoy to help you with your technique.

When racing in a triathlon, in most cases you will be provided a swim cap for your particular swim wave. And you will only have to bring your goggles and, if allowed, your wet suit.

A wet suit is a bit trickier, especially for women, as your body shape is very different from men's. However, what we have found with the huge growth of women in the sport is that most companies now have wet suits specifically for women. They tend to have shorter body lengths but longer arms and legs, and tend to have more room through the hips and chest. For some women's body types and physiques, a men's wet suit is a better fit.

A great way to find the best-fitting wet suit is to go to your local triathlon or running shop that caters to triathletes and try them on. Each brand is different, and a good fitter can help you find the right one. It should feel snug when you try it on but not so tight you cannot get it off. If the shop you go to only sells one brand and you aren't satisfied, try another local shop or order one on online. Be cautious though, because you cannot test a wet suit in the water and then return it. You can usually only try it on.

Another option is a wet-suit rental. Most triathlon and running shops now rent wet suits, which offers a great way to determine if that brand will fit you. You can rent it and take it to the local pool or open water to try it. We recommend you only swim for about 10 to 15 minutes in an indoor pool when wearing a wet suit to avoid overheating. Trying it in an outdoor pool or open water is best.

Cycling Equipment

Here is where it all starts to fall apart for most women, and truth be told, most men too. Selecting the best fitted bike and actually being comfortable on the bike, can be tricky. The two are not always synonymous. Issues ranging from the comfort of the bike seat to confidence in riding with clipless pedals can be a huge source of frustration and, quite frankly, fear.

Let's start with selecting a bike that works best for you. If you are new to the sport of triathlon and cycling, we suggest getting a comfortable road bike to start. It is the safest and most comfortable way to learn to ride for a beginner. If you are a competitive athlete and you know that you will want a triathlon-specific bike one year into the sport, you might as well start with a triathlon bike. The difference between a road bike and a triathlon bike is the geometry of the frame, the latter having steeper angles. A triathlon bike is less stable and requires better bike-handling skills than a road bike.

Another significant difference between men and women in this area is size. Most women are smaller than men and require a more compact frame, which in itself can be less stable when you move toward a triathlon bike. So consider your size (i.e., height and weight) and your ability before deciding on which type of bike to get, then consult with a few different bike shops before selecting one that will work best for you. Most bike shops only sell a few select brands and thus, for obvious reasons, push those brands. That is fine, but make sure you are comfortable with the ones they have.

We recommend you do a little research up front. First, make sure the bike shop has a very good reputation for fitting and service and is willing to help you learn some of the basics, like fixing a flat tire. In our experience, a good bike shop, with staff that provides these services, accounts for a lot more than price in selecting your bike. Additionally, a proper fit on a less expensive bike is better than having the most expensive bike if it doesn't fit you properly.

If you are less than 5 feet tall, you may have trouble finding a popular bike with the proper frame size. Often the smallest frame in a standard bike is 51 inches. If you are shorter than 5 feet 2 inches, you may want to consider a women-specific-design bike that has smaller overall dimensions and may have a smaller wheel size (650c vs. 700c). We recommend you try both types of bikes and ride them before you make your final decision. Go to the bike shop and be prepared to spend a couple of hours trying out bikes.

We always tell our athletes to learn the basics of their bikes and, most important, to know how to change a flat tire! It will happen to you on the roads and you must be prepared to change it. The bike is a very basic piece of equipment, and if you just know a few things about it, you will be better equipped when something goes wrong.

A bike is made up of several components, starting with the frame, componentry, pedals, and wheels. Other essential nonattached parts are bike shoes, cleats, and a helmet.

The basic frame in a road bike is made of aluminum or carbon fiber, the latter being lighter in weight but more expensive. Next come the two wheels, which are usually 700 cm and can have either tubular (which means it has no tube inside) or clincher tires (does have a tube inside). If you are a small or petite woman with a women-specific design, you may have a bike frame that comes with 650c wheels, and they can have tubular or clincher tires on those wheels as well. We recommend clinchers for newbies as they are much easier for changing a flat.

The other expensive parts to a bike are the components. The components are made up of the brakes, the shifters, and the front and rear derailleur. Most bikes come with a particular set of componentry that are commensurate with the price of the bike. The more expensive a bike, the more expensive the components.

In addition to the componentry, you will have to buy bike shoes and cleats, as well as clipless pedals. If you use clipless pedals, make sure you replace your cleats at least once per year as they do wear out. It is very important to avoid getting your cleats stuck in the pedals or breaking during a race. You could also use platform pedals. These are platforms that you use with your sneakers, and many beginners use them to start. With that said, though, if you can, we recommend you try clipless pedals as they do make for better riding.

If you have a triathlon bike, you probably have aero bars already. These are the bars attached to your handlebars on which you rest your forearms on the pads as you ride to reduce drag. They are used in the Tour de France during time trials (i.e., solo riding). They can be great, but unless you are comfortable on your bike, we recommend waiting to put aero bars on it.

Lastly, there's the bike seat. The dreaded bike seat! We can't tell you the complaints we get from women about the bike seat. It can be a troubling issue, from causing chafing to hard cysts forming in the labia to infections. Our experience with women has been wide ranging. So, if you are having an issue, you are not alone. The good news is that today there are many more women-specific bike seats that are designed to fit a woman's anatomy. For instance, some women-specific seats have a central cutout and wider rear seat as women's sit bones are typically wider than men's. It seems logical and it is tempting to get a saddle with lots of squishy gel, but these saddles are not as comfortable as they look. The gel moves and can pinch, and cheap gel often breaks down quickly. Saddles that offer firm support where you need it are better in the long run.

However, another key component is proper bike fit. If not done properly, it can cause you to have discomfort with the bike seat, although that may not be the issue. There is a bit of discomfort when you first start to ride, but once you get accustomed to it, it should dissipate and you will have normal pressure. The best bike seat is one you don't notice when you get on the bike.

A lot of manufacturers now have programs where you can use a demo seat and try a few before purchasing one. This is a great program, and if you are having issues with your bike seat, you may want to consider it.

To help you learn the basics of your bike, on the next page you will find a photo of Mel's bike with all the parts labeled. We seriously recommend you study this and try to learn these parts and components on your own bike. You will feel a lot more comfortable when you go to your local bike shop to purchase your first bike or to get your existing bike repaired or for maintenance.

Speaking of maintenance, we recommend you bring your bike in for maintenance at least once but ideally twice per year. Usually, you will want to do this before your first race of the season but well in advance—not three days before the race, but at least one to two weeks before your first race. You should allow for sufficient time to ride your bike after it has received maintenance to make sure nothing is out of whack.

And of course, don't forget a helmet! That's a must!

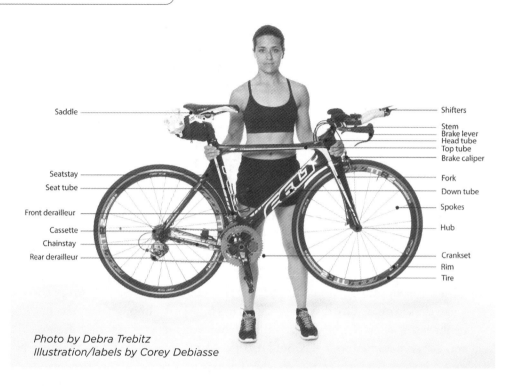

Saddle
Shifters
Stem
Brake lever
Head tube
Top tube
Brake caliper
Seatstay
Fork
Seat tube
Down tube
Front derailleur
Spokes
Cassette
Hub
Chainstay
Rear derailleur
Crankset
Rim
Tire

Photo by Debra Trebitz
Illustration/labels by Corey Debiasse

An IronFit Moment

How to Change a Flat Tire

We remember twenty-plus years ago when we got our first real bikes and the bike shop told us to just come in if we ever got a flat and they would fix it. We thought that was great—how nice of them! We quickly learned in most cases you are out for a ride when you get a flat tire and not within walking distance of the bike shop. That was our first mistake. Then, we thought we could just call one of our siblings or Mel's mom to come pick us up. Another mistake, as oftentimes, friends and family are not around when you need them. So, the moral of the story . . . learn to change a flat tire—it is easy if you practice. Most bike shops will even offer a quick one-hour demonstration for new riders, so take advantage of that usually free service. If that option is not available, you can always find an online video demonstration or try our instructions here.

1. Make sure you have all the necessary tools: replacement tube, pump or CO2 cartridge, tire levers, and stem extender if you have deep rim wheels with you in a pack attached to your bike.

2. Move off to the side of the road and take off the wheel of the tire you need to change. If it is the rear tire, shift the bike into the smallest cog of your cassette. And then open the brakes by pulling the release to allow the tire to slide through.

3. Then, standing on the non-chain side, flip the quick release skewer to the open position.

4. Grab the top tube of the bike and lift the rear wheel off the ground. The wheel should fall out of the dropouts.

5. While holding the top tube, take your other hand and press your finger down on the tab of the derailleur, which will cause slack in the chain. Move the frame away from your body so the chain falls off the rear cog set and frees the wheel from the bike.

6. Holding the wheel upright, align one of your levers with a spoke and insert the scoop end under the bead or edge of the tire, then hook the other end to the spoke.

7. Take your other lever about 3 inches from there and insert it scoop end under the bead or edge and begin to push the lever around the tire until it comes off the rim completely on one side while the other side remains in the rim. If the tire is old, you can usually do this with just your hands.

8. Then, pull the valve of the stem of the tube through the hole and remove the old tube, discarding it in your back pocket or far from the new tube to avoid mixing them up.

9. Make sure you inflate the old tube to see what caused the flat. It could be a "snakebite" or glass or debris that punctured a hole in the tube. Examine both the inside and outside of the tire itself as well for glass or debris. Rub your finger under the inside rim of the tire to check for glass or debris.

10. Take your new tube and open the valve before you blow a little air in it to slightly inflate it. This will give it a little more shape and make it easier to put back in the tire.

11. Then take the valve stem and insert it back in the hole through the rim and begin to feed the tube back under the tire.

12. Then with both hands starting at the valve and going in opposite directions toward each other, insert the tire under the rim. It will get more difficult to get the tire back under the rim the farther you get away from the valve. If you can't push that last few inches of tire under the rim, use one of your tire levers to get it over the rim and back in place. Just be careful not to pop the tube with your lever.

13. Inflate the tire before putting the wheel back on the bike using the specified tire PSI indicated on the rim of the tire (usually 100 to 110 psi for most tires).

14. Then, place the wheel back into the wheel drop-outs and place the chain on the smallest cog on the cassette. Hold the quick-release lever in the open position while tightening the nut on the chain side. The lever should be tight enough to pull off with two fingers but not one.

15. Last, close your brake release and spin the wheel to make sure it is not rubbing against the brake pad, and engage your right brake, which controls your rear brake, to make sure it stops the wheel.

Running

Now to a much easier sport in terms of equipment. After getting done with the whole bike thing, running seems quite simple. Go to your local running store and get fitted for a pair of running shoes. If you have orthotics, be sure to bring them with you for testing with the new sneakers. Also, if you have orthotics, you should get a neutral sneaker because the orthotics are already compensating for any issues you have.

We recommend tracking the mileage on your running shoes and changing them before you reach about 500 miles on them (or about sixty to eighty hours). Also, if you are a heavy runner, you may have to change them more often. It's also a good idea to have two pairs that you alternate with every other run.

Do you need orthotics? Do you have chronic injuries that may be helped by getting orthotics . . . maybe, maybe not? We recommend seeking the advice from an orthopedist, podiatrist, chiropractor, and/or physical therapist who has expertise with athletes, specifically runners and triathletes. If you are not having issues from an injury perspective, you probably do not need orthotics, so do not just get them because someone recommends them. We like to say, "If it ain't broke, don't fix it."

Heart Rate Monitors

As all of our cycling and running training is based on heart rate and time and we highly recommend you get yourself a heart rate monitor. It will be the best piece of gadgetry you own, as it will help you to train properly and give you feedback as to your exertion and fitness level. You can have the basic heart rate monitor that gives heart rate, time, and chronograph, or a more sophisticated one that also gives pace via GPS. Either one is fine.

The heart rate monitor has a chest strap and a wristband watch that you can wear in both training and racing. A common complaint we get from women is that the strap does not stay in place or causes chafing. To avoid this issue, make sure the strap is tight enough around your chest just under your breasts. If you experience chafing, use Body Glide or Vaseline in the chafing areas before you put it on. Or try one of the new wrist monitors that do not require a chest strap.

And you should realize, too, that as good as these gadgets are, they are not 100 percent perfect. Oftentimes you will get a misreading on the monitor and it may take a few miles before your heart rate monitor starts to register. Try wetting the strap at the contact points. And lastly, the GPS on these gadgets that track pace and distance is pretty far from 100 percent and that is a fact. We typically find the recorded distance is more than the distance ran, which then also throws off the pace. It is still best to learn and understand your pace manually by using your watch on a track or measure course.

Once you have determined your heart rate zones as described in Chapter 9, you will be already to put this gadget to use.

Training and Racing Clothing

With the huge growth of women's participation in triathlon, so goes the growth of triathlon-specific and women-specific clothing companies, which provide far superior clothing than even five years ago. It is a great thing. When we started in the sport twenty-plus years ago, we basically shared the same clothing because there was no difference.

If you are just getting into the sport, consider yourself lucky. You have many options to find biking shorts, helmets, and one- and two-piece triathlon racing suits specifically made for women.

We recommend you race in either a one-piece or two-piece triathlon suit. For larger-breasted women, you want to consider a suit that has a built-in bra or wear a sports bra that fits under your triathlon suit.

A couple of things to consider when getting a triathlon suit are the type of material and if it will cause you chafing or irritation. The second thing is whether you want an easy-to-remove suit for ease of using a port-a-john, if and when necessary. Practice with both a one- and two-piece in training and find which one works best for you.

In a triathlon racing suit, the bike pad is usually a lot smaller and thinner than in regular biking shorts, so again make sure you give it a try in training. The thinner pad will dry quicker since you will be wearing it under your wet suit.

A few other clothing issues to consider are socks and caps. Most triathletes will bike and run during a race wearing socks and either a visor or cap, since by the time you get to the run portion of the race, the sun is usually in full force.

One thing we have learned over the years is that triathlon is a petri dish for any new gadgetry, from bikes to wireless power meters, and for some causes great consternation. Just a little story to help you realize it is not about the bike, it's about the training.

Many years ago, we went out to California to do a cycling camp with world-class gold medal cyclist John Howard. Neither of us knew much about our bikes and could barely put them back together after we had removed the seat, pedals, and wheels to pack them and bring them with us on the plane. With a little help from the mechanic, we managed. However, there were some really experienced cyclists there with some bikes we had never seen before and with a price tag we could not imagine. When it came down to the last day, we all did a time trial on our bikes for a little friendly competition. Surprisingly, Don had the second-best finish time and was riding the least expensive bike. So, take it from us, beyond the basics of equipment, focus on your training and technique and you will see great results.

This chapter presents the fifth of seven motivating profiles of an inspiring female triathlete.

ATHLETE SUCCESS STORY:
JUDI GERMANO

Judi Germano is a busy attorney who has been married for over fifteen years and has two children. Despite a busy career and family responsibilities, Judi has also taken on the title "triathlete" in the past year.

Judi completed two Standard Distance triathlons and a Half Iron-Distance triathlon in her very first year. Judi is proud of these accomplishments, especially as she had to overcome the doubt and discouragement of some negative people around her who told her she was "foolish to try." Well, if anything, that was just fuel for Judi's motivational fire, and she enjoyed a very successful first year as a triathlete.

Triathlon was always a dream of Judi's because she loved cycling and thought it would be really cool to do all three sports. But she felt triathlon was something for "real athletes" and not for her. As life went on and Judi found herself juggling career and family, the dream of triathlon seemed even further out of reach.

But as is often the case, it just takes one unforeseen event to trigger change and to set us on a new journey. For Judi this moment came when she was persuaded to enter a Tough Mudder competition with work friends. While it was a great challenge, Judi completed the race and something was awakened inside of her. The fire was lit and she began running, in addition to cycling, and also started taking swim lessons. Once her swim ability and confidence caught up a bit with her cycling and running, Judi took the next step and signed up for her first triathlon. Now after three successful triathlons in her first year of competition, the sky is the limit.

Amazingly, in addition to being a successful attorney, wife, and mother, Judi is a competitive athlete. How does she do it? Judi says that it's all about effective time management. "I deal with it two ways: 1) Make it count, and 2) resist the guilt. I do my best to focus on what I am doing at that moment and give it my all, whether time with family, tasks at work, or training. I make a detailed daily schedule of what I need to accomplish, where I need to be when, and how I will get it all done, and (since flexibility also is essential) I revise that as needed. So when I am training, I can't feel guilty about family or work because it is the time I carved out to train . . . and I also don't want to squander a workout by just going through the motions because I know it is a trade-off against all the other things on the list. So whatever it is I am doing, I aim to 'make it count.' It also helps immensely to have an awesome and experienced coach who sets my workouts so I can maximize time-efficient training, and keeps me motivated and accountable when I otherwise would short-change (or completely drop!) my health goals due to everything else I am juggling."

Judi Germano is indeed a wonderful example of making it count.

CHAPTER 6

Eight Essential Training Sessions

We can do anything we want
if we stick to it long enough.

—Helen Keller, author, activist, and lecturer

O f course it is not just about swimming, cycling, and running every day and then showing up on race day to compete. There are eight specific types of workouts that should optimally be included in an athlete's program to maximize training and a specific way each of these sessions should be executed.

These eight workouts are not the training program itself but the basic building blocks for designing a perfect training program. Each workout has a specific purpose and then is properly grouped together with the other sessions to maximize the desired training benefit. Anything less than this approach amounts to what we refer to as "junk training."

While these workouts will be tweaked and adjusted slightly depending on which triathlon distance the athlete is preparing for, these sessions are all used in the training programs in this book. The Sprint and Standard Distance, Half Iron-Distance, Full Iron-Distance, and Off-Season Training Programs presented in Chapters 10, 11, 12, and 16 use these eight important training sessions and perfectly builds them into each program to maximize the athlete's training benefit.

Here are the eight key workouts:
1. Transition sessions (aka bricks)
2. The long run
3. The long ride
4. Higher-intensity bike sessions
5. Higher-intensity run sessions

6. High-rpm-technique spins
7. The IronFit Swim Training Approach: intervals, drills, open water, and Masters
8. Strategic rest days/slide days

We will clearly define each of these eight sessions in full detail and do so in a straightforward and easily understandable way. We will explain what each session's duration should be, how frequently it should be completed, and at what level of training intensity.

Most important these workouts are fun. Training does not have to be drudgery. We design these sessions to be both highly productive and highly enjoyable.

While men and women athletes both do these types of workouts, the priority of these workouts differs between men and woman. In other words, most women can benefit by focusing more on some of the eight key training sessions than others. We explain these secrets and show you exactly what you need to do to maximize the benefit of their training time.

Following is a discussion of each of the Eight Essential Training Sessions.

Transition Sessions (aka Bricks)

Transition sessions are sessions that involve two or more sports, each separated by a quick change from the gear of one sport to the other. The most common example of a brick session is a "bike-to-run brick." In this session we ride for a specific amount of time at a specific level of intensity and then stop, quickly change from our cycling gear into our running gear, and then run for a specific amount of time at a specific level of intensity.

A typical example of a bike-to-run brick is as follows:

Trans: 45 min. Z2 Bike (QC) 15 min. Z2 Run

In this simple brick session, we start off by cycling for 45 minutes in a Z2 heart rate (**Note:** We will discuss heart rates in Chapter 9, but for now it is only important to know that this means a moderate intensity). As soon as we complete the 45 minutes of cycling, we quickly change from our cycling gear into our running gear (**Note:** A good target is within 5 minutes) and then run for 15 minutes at a Z2 heart rate (moderate intensity).

Although very typical, this is just one example of a brick session. Bricks can range in terms of duration and intensity level, as well as the sports involved. For example, you could do a swim-to-bike brick. As you will see in the training programs in this book, we suggest brick sessions as short as 45 minutes and as long as seven hours, depending on many factors, including the distance of the race for which one is training and the experience level of the athlete.

Why is the bike-to-run brick such an important training session in the sport of triathlon? It's because running immediately after cycling is one of the most challenging demands that triathlon puts on our bodies, and brick sessions help to prepare our bodies to excel at this challenge.

The Long Run

We consider long runs to be runs of 90 minutes or more and completed at a relatively moderate aerobic heart rate (Z1 to Z2; see Chapter 9).

The long run builds running endurance and aerobic strength, which is especially important in triathlon as the run always comes after the swim and bike. In fact, the most common mistake with long runs is that athletes complete them at too high of an intensity. This defeats the purpose of this session and also is risky for injury.

As coaching great Peter Gavuzzi famously said, "Three hours slow is better than two hours fast."

There are important training benefits that can only be achieved by doing this session properly. The key is to properly structure the long runs at just the right duration, intensity, and frequency, within an overall training program.

As you will see in the training programs in this book, the actual length of the long runs will vary depending on the triathlon distance for which an athlete is training.

The Long Ride

We consider long rides to be rides of two hours or more, but unlike the long runs, they are completed at a variety of intensities, depending on the triathlon distance for which the athlete is training. Most athletes spend over half of a triathlon on their bikes, so it's not surprising these sessions are so important.

The training programs in this book include long rides from two hours all of the way up to six hours, depending on the racing distance being covered. While most of these rides are completed at a moderate level of intensity (heart rate Z2), some portions of these rides are often completed at high intensity (heart rate Z4).

Since these are typically the longest training sessions of the week, they are generally scheduled for weekends when most athletes have time to complete them. But for those who actually have more time during the week, we have suggested approaches like the "mom shift" to adapt the training programs to you and your lifestyle.

When possible, we often like to plan for the long ride on the day before the long run, as this best simulates a racing situation where you will begin the final running portion of the races on legs already tired from the bike.

For this same reason, some of the programs combine the long ride and the transition (aka "brick") sessions together into a long brick. This provides one of the most challenging training sessions.

Higher-Intensity Bike Sessions

The two basic types of higher-intensity bike sessions are "Z4 Inserts" and "Z4 Repeats." The following is an example of a Z4 Insert session:

60 min. Z2 (at 45 min., insert 10 min. Z4)

In this 60-minute session the athlete cycles for the first 45 minutes in Z2 (moderate intensity). We will discuss heart rates zones in greater detail in Chapter 9, but for now the important point to know is that Z2 represents a fairly moderate intensity level, while Z4 represents a high-intensity effort level. At the 45-minute point in the ride, the athlete increases her intensity up to heart rate Z4 (higher intensity) by cycling faster. At exactly 10 minutes after the athlete first started trying to increase her heart rate up to Z4, the athlete will lower her intensity and will complete the remainder of the 60 minutes (which in this situation equals 5 minutes) in heart rate zone 2 (moderate intensity).

The following is an example of a Z4 Repeat session:

60 min. Z2 (at 10 min., insert 5 x 4 min. Z4 @ 2 min. spin)

In this 60-minute session, the athlete cycles for the first 10 minutes in Z2 (moderate intensity). At the 10-minute point in the ride, the athlete increases her intensity up to heart rate Z4 (higher intensity) by cycling faster. At exactly 4 minutes after the athlete first started trying to increase her heart rate up to Z4, the athlete will lower her intensity to an easy spin for 2 minutes. The athlete will repeat this sequence of 4 minutes "hard" followed by 2 minutes "easy" for a total of 5 repetitions. Once the 5th repetition has been completed, the athlete will complete the remainder of the 60 minutes (which in this situation equals 20 minutes) in heart rate zone 2 (moderate intensity).

An important variation of the Z4 Repeat session is the Hill Repeat Session. These sessions not only help to develop great cycling strength, they also help prepare athletes to race well on hilly courses, as well as flatter courses.

The following is an example of a Z4 Hill Repeat Session:

60 min. Z2 (at 10 min., insert 10 x 2 min. Z4 Hill
Repeat @ spin back down)

In this 60-minute session, the athlete cycles for the first 10 minutes in Z2 (moderate intensity), planning to arrive at the base of a hill right at the 10-minute mark. At the 10-minute point in the ride, the athlete cycles up the hill fast enough to increase her heart rate to Z4 (higher intensity). At exactly 2 minutes after the athlete first started riding up the hill, she safely and cautiously turns her bike around and spins easily down the hill, returning to the base of the hill starting point. Once she arrives at the base of the hill, she safely and cautiously turns her bike around and again cycles back up the hill in a Z4 heart rate (higher intensity). The athlete will repeat this sequence of up and down the hill for a total of 10 repetitions. Once the 10th repetition has been completed, the athlete will complete the remainder of the 60 minutes in heart rate Z2 (moderate intensity).

The time of this final portion will vary depending on how long it took the athlete to spin back down the hill after each uphill portion. In general, depending on the steepness of the hill, we find that it typically takes the athletes two-thirds as long to spin easily down the hill as it took them to cycle at higher intensity up the hill.

Higher-Intensity Run Sessions

The two basic types of higher-intensity run sessions are "Z4 Inserts" and "Z4 Repeats." The following is an example of a Z4 Insert session:

60 min. Z2 (at 45 min., insert 10 min. Z4)

In this 60-minute session, the athlete runs for the first 45 minutes in Z2 (moderate intensity). We will discuss heart rates zones in greater detail in Chapter 9, but for now the important point to know is that Z2 represents a fairly moderate intensity level, while Z4 represents a high-intensity effort level. At the 45-minute point in the run, the athlete increases her intensity up to heart rate Z4 (higher intensity) by running faster. At exactly 10 minutes after the athlete first started trying to increase her heart rate up to Z4, the athlete will lower her intensity and will complete the remainder of the 60 minutes (which in this situation equals 5 minutes) in heart rate zone 2 (moderate intensity).

The following is an example of a Z4 Repeat session:

60 min. Z2 (at 10 min., insert 7 x 3 min. Z4 @ 1.5 min. jog)

In this 60-minute session, the athlete runs for the first 10 minutes in Z2 (moderate intensity). We will discuss heart rates zones in greater detail in Chapter 9, but for now the important point to know is that Z2 represents a fairly moderate intensity level, while Z4 represents a high-intensity effort level. At the 10-minute point in the run, the athlete increases her intensity up to heart rate Z4 (higher intensity) by running faster. At exactly 3 minutes after the athlete first started trying to increase her heart rate up to Z4, the athlete will lower her intensity to an easy jog for 1.5 minutes. The athlete will repeat this sequence of 3 minutes "hard" followed by 1.5 minutes "easy" for a total of 7 repetitions. Once the 7th repetition has been completed, the athlete will complete the remainder of the 60 minutes (which in this situation equals 18.5 minutes) in heart rate zone 2 (moderate intensity).

Similar to the higher-intensity cycling sessions, it's also possible to structure Z4 Repeats as Hill Repeats. In general, however, we typically don't utilize Running Hill Repeats for most athletes. These tend to be less beneficial for triathlon than cycling Hill Repeats and they are more risky for injury. The risk-versus-reward equation is not as attractive as it is for Cycling Hill Repeats, and a triathlete can build her hill-running abilities just as well by including hilly courses in her running workouts.

High-RPM-Technique Spins

High-rpm spins are cycling sessions where we spin the pedals at a relatively high cadence of about 100 to 105 revolutions per minute (rpm) but we do so at a low-intensity effort level with a heart rate of Z1. To do this we must be in a very easy gear (low resistance) to allow us to spin the pedals quickly while keeping our heart rate down at a fairly low level.

Most athletes don't realize the great value of these high-rpm spins because of the comfortably low heart rate. In typical "triathlete logic," if it doesn't hurt, it cannot possibly have any benefit. But of course, this is not true. In fact, these sessions have two major benefits.

First, high-rpm spins help us develop good cycling form. We want to be spinning the pedals in a circular pattern, not mashing them down and pulling them up. "Spinning circles" is the most efficient way to cycle. The important point, however, is that it is very difficult to achieve a high cadence like 100 to 105 rpm unless you are spinning circles. So, if you find that you have difficulty spinning your pedals at this high of a cadence, this may be an especially important training session for you. But even if you are very accomplished at spinning circles at a high cadence, these sessions are very beneficial in building and maintaining good cycling form.

Secondly, these are excellent sessions for recovery. The combination of the high cadence and low resistance helps legs to recover and freshen up for the next day's training. As you will see in the training programs in this book, when these sessions are included, they are usually positioned among the other workouts of the week where they can maximize this benefit.

The IronFit Swim Training Approach: Intervals, Drills, Open Water, and Masters

One of the greatest assets a triathlete can have available to her is a convenient local Masters Swim program. It makes swim progress so much easier compared to having to swim on your own. Most programs will meet several times a week, so you can select the two or three weekly times that fit your schedule best. Then, all you need to do is show up on time just like you would for any other appointment, and everything pretty much takes care of itself.

This may be a slight exaggeration, but in an ideal program there will be a good coach on deck who will design fun and challenging workouts and also offer feedback from time to time regarding your swim progress. Many programs today even specialize in triathletes and open-water swimmers, so the workouts are heavily weighted toward freestyle.

But this is a nice-to-have, not a need-to-have, specialized program, and a general program with plenty of stroke work can be very beneficial as well. In fact, many swimmers find that they progress more by training in all four strokes, even though they still do the majority in freestyle.

Most Masters Swim sessions have swim workouts of one hour, which allows you to fairly easily get two to three quality hours of swimming in weekly.

Another great benefit of Masters Swim programs is that they are packed with motivation. Many find swimming alone to be boring, but swimming in a lane of enthusiastic and motivated swimmers like you will make your swim time fun and motivating.

But what if you don't have a Masters Swim program available to you? No worries, we have included sixty-six swim sessions in this book and each training program shows you exactly when to use each session. We also provide drills and other tips and advice on swimming to help you to build your swim even without a Masters program. All you will need to do is to find a local pool with "open lap swim" times and you are good to go.

Finally, whether you are swimming with a Masters program or using the swim sessions we suggest in this book, it is also suggested that you practice swimming in open water as well. And if it is likely you will be racing in a wet suit, you should practice in your wet suit at least occasionally. Swimming in open water and in a wet suit feels much different than swimming in a pool, so we need time to feel comfortable in the open water.

If there are open-water races near you, these are great opportunities not only to become comfortable swimming in the open water but to get actual racing experience as well.

You can also just swim practice sessions in the open water, but please play it safe and only do this in the presence of a competent lifeguard.

Strategic Rest Days/Slide Days

Just the mention of the phrase "rest day" makes many "type A" triathletes cringe. But rest days are absolutely essential to optimizing our training. Our bodies absolutely need the proper amount of time to recover and absorb the good benefits of our training. Many athletes cannot get their minds around this and they are continually frustrated by injury and performance stagnation. The rest day should be viewed like any other key workout. We often jokingly refer to it with our coached athletes as "the non-workout workout."

There are one or two weekly rest days strategically built into all of the training programs in this book. We say "strategically" because they are placed among the other workouts in the week at a point where they will prove most beneficial.

Now here's the secret to most effectively using rest days: Instead of just referring to them as "rest days," we will designate them as "rest days/slide days." In other words, use them to slide your rest days forward by one day or back by one day to help your training schedule to work better around your overall schedule in a particular week.

For example, Monday is your rest day/slide day, but you find out that you have a commitment coming up this week on Tuesday that will prevent you from training that day. To remedy this, simply slide Tuesday's training session forward to Monday and designate Tuesday as your rest day for that week.

All of the workouts are designed in a specific order for good reason, so we want to avoid "flipping" them during the week if possible. Instead, if something comes up and you cannot get a planned workout in on the day for which it is planned, simply slide your rest day/slide day forward or back one day to accommodate the situation. This allows you to get all of your training sessions in while keeping them in the order in which they were intended and still get the benefit of your rest days.

The training programs presented in this book use these Eight Essential Training Sessions and build them into each program to maximize the athlete's training benefit. We have designed these programs in a way to totally eliminate the guesswork. Just follow the program each day, and enjoy the challenge and the journey.

Following is the sixth of seven motivating profiles of an inspiring female triathlete.

ATHLETE SUCCESS STORY:
MARIENNE HILL-TREADWAY

Marienne Hill-Treadway is an executive in the fashion industry in New York City. So she has all of the usual challenges of being a female triathlete, plus she has a high-stress, fast-paced career and a challenging daily commute from her suburban home. Despite this, Marienne has successfully competed in triathlons each year for more than five years and enjoys the Standard Distance (aka Olympic Distance) the most.

As with many triathletes, Marienne started out as a runner, but after an injury (in her case, a stress fracture) she was attracted to the cross-training nature of triathlon. While recovering from the fracture, she started spin classes and some swim lessons, and before long Marienne was a triathlete.

Professional women have their own set of challenges when it comes to being a competitive athlete. As an executive in the fashion industry, Marienne gets up early each weekday to squeeze in as much as 90 minutes of training before she commutes into New York City. As Marienne points out, the entire process is very challenging, "The hair, the heels, and the makeup . . . it all takes time." But the rewards are even greater than the challenges, and that is why she does it.

Marienne has successfully dealt with many of the menopause-related challenges that most female athletes either are or will be confronted with. She developed a stress fracture in her femur due to a low-bone-density issue relating to premenopause. This then led to other related health issues that frustratingly took two years and multiple doctors to sort out.

Then, as soon as she thought she had that under control, at age 51 she developed full-blown menopause. She suffered frequent sleepless nights due to night sweats. She would then wake up tired in the mornings, making morning training especially challenging.

Marienne's best tips for women entering triathlon include the following:

- Get a complete health checkup to make sure there are no issues.
- Be patient and take it one day at a time.
- Be super-organized.
- Get plenty of sleep.
- Make sure you have two sets of cosmetics and beauty bags—one at home and one for your gym bag.
- Marry someone who will be your biggest fan!

CHAPTER 7

Functional Muscle Strength and Core for the Female Triathlete

*Only the weak attempts to accomplish what
he knows he can already achieve.*

—Stella Juarez, diet and nutrition expert

One of the key elements to being a successful triathlete is managing the multitude of aspects of triathlon training. This includes the obvious swimming, biking, and running, but another component that is very important is functional muscle and core strength. Without them, your success in triathlon will be limited. This is much truer for female triathletes than their male counterparts. Women have a smaller amount of muscle mass to begin with and typically begin to lose muscle mass and function in their early thirties.

After coaching female triathletes for many years and from our own experience in the sport, we know that as we age, muscle mass and function become more and more important in staying healthy and avoiding injury.

Two other often overlooked areas that require some attention are a solid warm-up routine that can be used before training and racing, and a concise stretching and flexibility routine to be used after a training session.

We understand that as an athlete becomes time-pressured, strengthening, warm-up, and stretching routines are usually the first things to be pushed aside in a training program. Although a warm-up and stretching can literally be done in 5 to 10 minutes before and after a workout and will provide great benefit to you in remaining healthy and injury-free, it is often overlooked along with the forever-ditched functional and core strength-training session.

If you could follow a three-season approach that would keep you strong and healthy while still maintaining that level of balance in your life, would you do it? Of course you would. Can you fit in one to two sessions of 15 to 20 minutes a week? The answer is probably yes.

Typically in the off-season, our nonracing months, we will bring our cardio hours down and this will allow us that extra time for core and strength training. We can focus on some areas of weakness that we may have experienced during the season and bring back better overall function and muscle strength.

So let's get started. We will lay out a three-season approach to our functional core and strength training beginning with our off-season program, then our preseason program, and then finish with our in-season maintenance program. So, wherever you are in your training, you can pick up with the appropriate program.

Let's start with a basic functional core and strength-training program that you can do two times per week for 15 to 20 minutes in the off-season. This program can be done at home or in the gym. It is meant to be a total body routine to help strengthen areas of weakness typically found in women and areas that need to be developed to perform better as a triathlete and to stay healthy and injury-free.

We start with ten exercises that we will perform on two separate days and preferably nonconsecutive days. We recommend, if possible, you perform these exercises in a circuit fashion, which means you do one set of each exercise through all of the exercises and then repeat two more times for a total of three circuits. This is the most efficient way to do the exercises.

It is best to read through the descriptions of all of the exercises to get a better understanding of how to perform them and their purposes before you begin.

Off-Season Exercises

Day One

1. Transverse Lunge with Row
2. Reverse Fly in Stork Position
3. Back Lunge with Overhead Reach
4. Push-Up with Hip Extension
5. Side Planks

Day Two

1. Side Lunge with Shoulder Press
2. Reverse Wood Chop with Cable or Stretch Cord
3. Push-Ups with Knee Tuck over Stability Ball
4. Front Lunge with Dumbbells
5. Torso Rotation with Medicine Ball

Day One: Off-Season

1. Transverse Lunge with Row

Functionality: To strengthen your glutes, hamstrings, quads, abductors, obliques, abs, shoulders, back, and arms.

Start in a standing position with a stretch cord (anchored to a door frame) in your right hand. Raise your arm straight and parallel to the floor in front of you while holding the stretch cord at shoulder height. Begin the exercise by taking a 45° step or lunge to your side with your right leg and simultaneously pulling back the stretch cord while keeping your arm parallel to the ground. Hold that position for 1 second and then return to the starting position. Repeat for the desired number of repetitions before switching to the other side. (See photos 1a and 1b.)

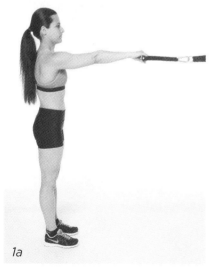
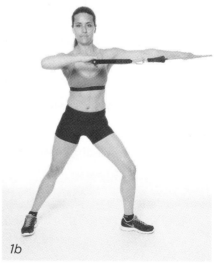

1a

1b

First progression: Same as above, except the lunging leg lands on a step.
Second progression: Same as above, except the lunging leg lands on a BOSU.
Sets/repetitions: Three sets of 10 to 12 each side.

2. Reverse Fly in Stork Position

Functionality: To strengthen your glutes, hamstrings, quads, abdominals, shoulders, deltoids, back, and arms.

Start in a standing position with a lightweight dumbbell in each hand. Begin by bringing one leg off the ground straight behind you in a stork position. Be sure your shoulder blades are depressed and pulled toward your spine as you raise your arms straight out to your sides by squeezing your shoulder blades together. Hold that position for 1 second, then return to the starting position. Split the desired numbered of repetitions on each leg.
First progression: Same as original exercise, except instead of performing the exercise simultaneously with both arms, alternate arms.
Second progression: Same as above, except begin the exercise by performing a one-leg squat and then raising your arms out to the sides as you return to the starting position. (See photos 2a and 2b.)
Sets/repetitions: Three sets of 10 to 12 total.

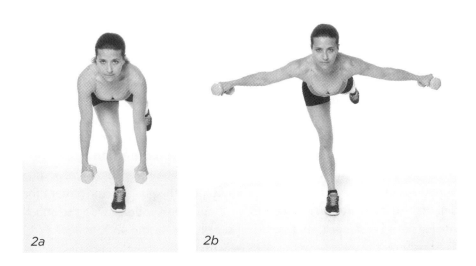

2a   2b

3. Back Lunge with Overhead Reach

Functionality: To strengthen your glutes, quads and obliques, abs, shoulders, and arms.

Start in a standing position with a heavier dumbbell in your left hand and lighter dumbbell in your right hand. Begin by taking a step back with your right leg into a lunge position as you simultaneously raise your right arm in an arching position with your palm facing up over your head. Hold the position for 1 second, then return to the starting position. Repeat the desired number of repetitions with that leg and arm and then switch weights in hands and repeat with opposite leg and arm. (See photo 3.)

First progression: Same as above, except begin the exercise by standing on a step and lunge back off the step with one foot.

Second progression: Same as above, except start by standing on a BOSU with one foot planted in the center and the other touching the side before you take a lunge back.

Sets/repetitions: Three sets of 10 to 12 each side.

4. Push-Up with Hip Extension

Functionality: To strengthen your chest, shoulders, arms, back, and core.

Begin with your knees bent on the floor and your hands a little wider than shoulder width apart. Pull your belly to your spine as you raise one leg straight back and parallel to the floor. Then perform a push-up by bringing your chest toward the floor as your elbows bend to a 90° angle. Press your body back up to the starting position and repeat the push-up movement for half of the desired number of repetitions. Reposition yourself with the opposite leg raised and repeat on that side. (See photos 4a and 4b.)

First progression: Perform the exercise with the leg straight and toes on the floor while the opposite leg is raised and straight.

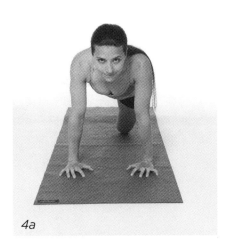

4a

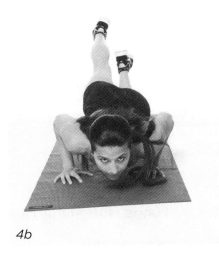

4b

Second progression: Perform the exercise the same as the first progression but with one foot on a raised step or bench to increase the difficulty while the raised leg remains off the step or bench.

Sets/repetitions: Three sets of 10 to 20 total.

5. Side Planks

Functionality: To strengthen your obliques, abdominals, core, and shoulders.

Start by lying on your side on the floor, with your upper body resting on your bent elbow under your shoulder and your other arm at your side. Draw in your belly and hold while raising your hip and torso off the floor, with weight on your forearm, until there is a straight line from your ankles to your head. Hold this position for up to 60 seconds. Once you can do that on both sides, then move to the first progression.

First progression: Same as the basic except raise your top arm straight up from your side and hold it there as you raise and lower your torso. (See photos 5a and 5b.)

Second progression: Same as basic exercise, except now raise one leg off the ground and hold for up to 60 seconds. Then repeat on the other side.

Repetition: Hold for up to 60 seconds / three sets of 10 to 15 each side (first progression only).

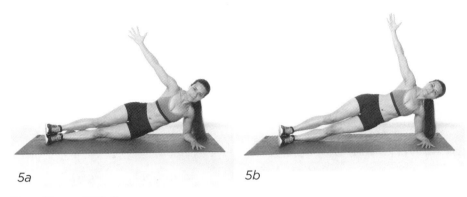

5a   5b

Day Two: Off-Season

1. Side Lunge with Shoulder Press

Functionality: To strengthen your glutes, hamstrings, abductors, quads, core, shoulders, and upper body.

Start in a standing position with feet about shoulder width apart and holding a dumbbell in each hand at shoulder height with palms facing inward. Begin by shifting your weight to your heels and engaging your abdominals. Then take a step to your right with your right leg shifting your weight to your right heel and pushing your hips back while your left leg remains straight. Both heels stay flat on the floor and toes are pointed forward. Simultaneously raise the dumbbells toward ceiling as you rotate your

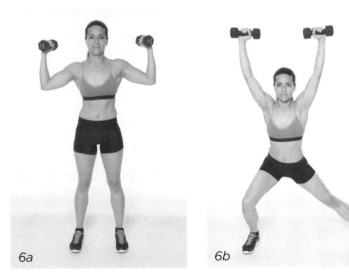

6a   6b

hands so your palms are facing forward as you reach a full lunge position. Split the desired number of repetitions between both legs. **Tip:** Avoid taking too big of a step by making sure the shinbone is aligned over your foot. (See photos 6a and 6b.)

First progression: Same as above, except begin the exercise by standing on a step and lunge off the step with one foot.

Second progression: Same as above, except start by standing on the BOSU with one foot planted in the center and the other touching the side before you lunge the other foot to the side.

Sets/repetitions: Three sets of 10 to 12 total.

2. Reverse Wood Chop with Cable or Stretch Cord

Functionality: To strengthen your back, shoulders, arms, glutes, and core.

Start by affixing a stretch cord to the bottom of a door frame or using a cable machine with a low row. Take hold of the stretch cord or cable with both hands, aligning your body parallel to the stretch cord or cable with feet beyond shoulder width so the cord is tight. Engage your abdominals and keep your arms straight as you pull the cord or cable across your torso to above your opposite shoulder. Hold that position for 1 second before returning to the starting position. (See photos 7a and 7b.) Repeat on the other side.

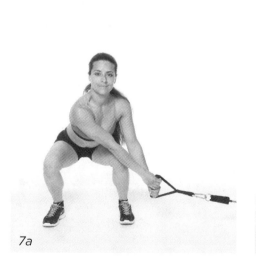
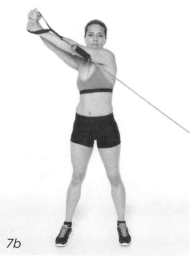

7a

7b

First progression: Same as above, except perform this exercise while kneeling on the floor with your knees about shoulder width apart.

Second progression: Same as above, except start by performing this exercise while standing on the BOSU. Begin with knees slightly bent to start as you pull the stretch cord or cable across your body and then straighten your legs as you bring it over your shoulder.

Sets/repetitions: Three sets of 10 to 12 each side.

3. Push-Ups with Knee Tuck over Stability Ball

Functionality: To strengthen your shoulders, chest, arms, back, abdominals, and core.

Start by lying flat on your stomach on a stability ball, with your arms out in front of you about shoulder width apart. Begin engaging your abdominals and walking your hands out from the ball until your shins are resting on the ball. Perform a push-up by bending at your elbows and bring your chest toward the floor. Extend back up, pull your knees toward your chest while engaging your abdominals, then extend back to the starting position. If combining these exercises is too much for you, roll back on the ball until you get to a position where you can do a push-up. Perform the push-up only until you can work up to the push-up with the ball at your shins, and then add back the knee tuck. (See photos 8a and 8b.)

First progression: Same as above, except after you perform the push-up, perform a pike instead of a knee tuck. To do this, keep your legs straight, engage your core and raise your butt toward the ceiling while keeping your legs straight, and bring your toes to the top of the ball.

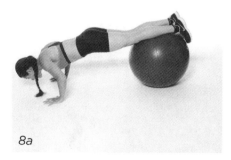

8a

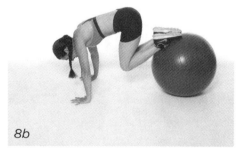

8b

Second progression: Same as first progression, except perform the knee tuck exercise with only one leg on the stability ball and the other raised off the stability ball.
Sets/repetitions: Three sets of 10 to 12.

4. Front Lunge with Dumbbells

Functionality: To strengthen your quads, glutes, hamstrings, shoulders, arms, and core.

Start in a standing position with your feet together with a dumbbell in each hand. Begin by taking a step forward, bringing the lunging leg quad parallel to the floor and the back leg slightly bent as you go onto your toe. Return to the starting position and repeat with the opposite leg. **Tip:** Avoid taking too big of a step by making sure to keep your knee aligned over your ankle. (See photo 9.)

First progression: Same as above, except perform a walking lunge with a 2-second hold on each leg.

Second progression: Same as above, except hold a medicine ball in your hands at chest height and lunge forward, rotating the medicine ball across your torso to the outside of the lunging leg to work your core and upper body. Return to the starting position and repeat with the opposite leg and rotate to the opposite side. Repeat for the desired number of repetitions.

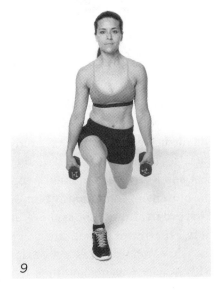

9

Sets/repetitions: Three sets of 10 to 15 each leg.

5. Torso Rotation with Medicine Ball

Functionality: To strengthen your glutes, hamstrings, abdominals, core, and obliques.

Start by sitting on a stability ball, holding a medicine ball in both hands. Walk your feet out from the stability ball as you lie on your back on the ball.

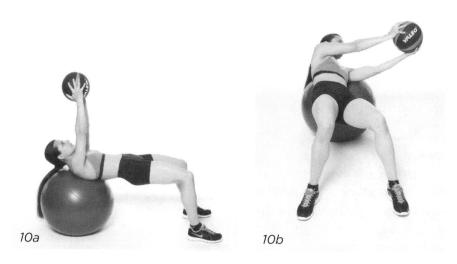

10a   10b

Keep your hips extended and knees bent, creating a straight line from your knees to your shoulders while your head remains elevated off the ball. Raise the medicine ball straight up from your chest with both hands and start the exercises by rotating the ball to one side while rolling onto your shoulder on that side. Keep your abdominals engaged as you rotate to the other side. Repeat the movement continuously from side to side. (See photos 10a and 10b.)

First progression: Same as above, but perform this exercise with a weight plate.

Sets/repetitions: Three sets of 20, alternating sides.

These ten exercises can be done for two to three months, progressing with heavier weights and then to the first and second progressions of the exercise.

When we are about two to three months out from our first race, we'll flip the switch and work on our dynamic power in our preseason. We'll take the number of exercises down to six to coincide with the increase in intensity in our training schedule.

Preseason Exercises

Day One

1. Side to Side Across BOSU with Medicine Ball
2. Mountain Climbers
3. Forward Lunge with Overhead Reach

Day Two

1. Jump Squats onto a Step or Box
2. Lunge Squat with Medicine Ball Rotation
3. Abdominals over Stability Ball with Medicine Ball

Day One

1. Side to Side Across BOSU with Medicine Ball

Functionality: To strengthen your glutes, hamstrings, quads, core, and arms.

Start this exercise by standing next to the BOSU with your right foot on the BOSU and the other foot off, while holding a medicine ball in your hands. Begin in a squat position and jump across the BOSU so your left foot lands on the top of the BOSU and your right on the floor. Your weight shifts to the leg on the BOSU as you land in the squat position. Repeat with a continuous side-to-side movement across the BOSU for the desired number of repetitions.

First progression: Same as above, but extend the medicine ball forward by bringing your arms straight out from your chest as your outer foot lands off the BOSU. Then, bring it back to your chest as you jump across and again extend it in front of you when your outer foot lands on the floor. (See photos 11a and 11b.)

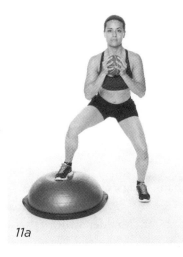
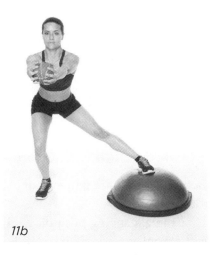

11a   11b

Second progression: Same as above, except holding a kettlebell with both hands and starting in a squat position, as you jump across the BOSU, bring the kettlebell straight out in front and then lower it between your legs as your outer foot lands on the floor. Repeat in a continuous movement as you go back and forth across the BOSU.

Sets: Three sets of 20 repetitions.

2. Mountain Climbers

Functionality: To strengthen your glutes, hamstrings, quads, core, back, and arms.

Start this exercise in a push-up position with arms straight and hands wider than your shoulders, legs straight and about shoulder width apart. Begin by bringing one knee forward without raising your hips and without touching the floor. Bring that leg back and repeat the movement with the opposite leg. This should be done in a continuous quick motion, alternating legs and holding your abdominals nice and tight. (See photos 12a and 12b.)

First progression: Same as above, except start with your hands on a raised step.

Second progression: Same as above, except start with your hands holding the sides of a BOSU with the flat side facing up.

Sets: Three sets of 10 to 15 repetitions each leg.

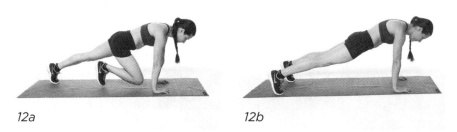

12a   *12b*

3. Forward Lunge with Overhead Reach

Functionality: To strengthen your glutes, hamstrings, quads, obliques, core, and arms.

Start in a standing position with feet about shoulder width apart and a light weight in your right hand. Begin by taking one step forward with

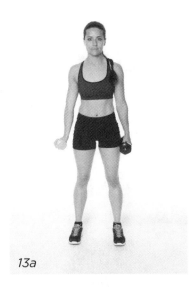

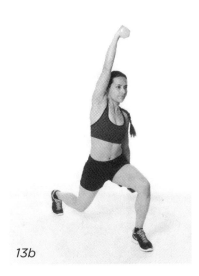

13a   13b

your left leg at a 45° angle and simultaneously bringing your right arm, with your palm facing up, over your head in an arching motion. Hold that position for 1 second, then return to the start position. Repeat this motion with the same leg and arm for the desired number of repetitions before switching the weight to your left hand and repeating the movement pattern with the opposite leg and arm.

First progression: Same as above, except add more difficulty by adding a heavier dumbbell in the lunge-side hand as well. (See photos 13a and 13b.)

Second progression: Increase the difficulty without using the dumbbells by performing a plyometric lunge. Take a step straight forward into a lunge position, bringing the knee of your back leg about 3 inches off the floor and keeping the other knee of your front leg over your ankle. Begin by jumping straight up and switching legs and landing back in that lunge position. Repeat the movement, alternating legs.

Sets: Three sets of 12 repetitions each leg.

Day Two

1. Jump Squats onto a Step or Box

Functionality: To strengthen glutes, hamstrings, quads, ankles, abs, core and balance.

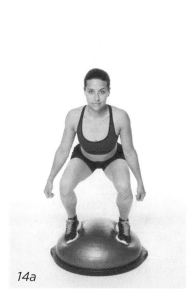
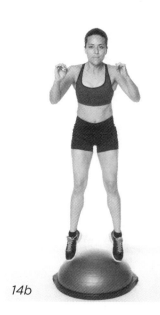

14a   14b

Start in a standing position with your feet about shoulder width apart in front of a step or box. With your arms at your sides, inhale and perform a deep squat. From the deep squat position, exhale and jump onto the step or box with both feet landing in a squat position. Step back off step and repeat the movement for the desired number of repetitions.

First progression: Same as above, except jump onto a BOSU, landing in a squat position.

Second progression: Start by standing on the BOSU. Perform a deep squat and jump by extending your legs, hips, and glutes straight up, then landing in a deep squat position back on the BOSU. Repeat that movement for the desired number of repetitions. (See photos 14a and 14b.)

Sets: Three sets of 15 to 20 repetitions.

2. Lunge Squat with Medicine Ball Rotation

Functionality: To strengthen glutes, hamstrings, quads, core, and arms.

Start in a lunge position holding a medicine ball to the side of the front leg. Begin by raising your back leg with bent knee forward and straight up while simultaneously bringing the medicine ball across your body toward the other side. Repeat for desired number of repetitions on that leg and then switch legs and repeat. (See photos 15a and 15b.)

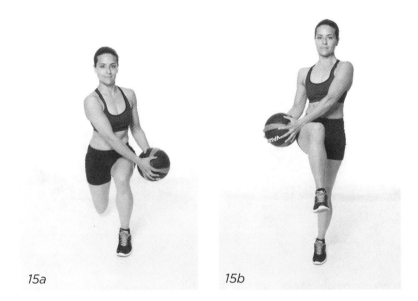

15a

15b

First progression: Same as above, except start standing with the forward leg on a step.

Second progression: Same as basic, except start standing with the forward leg on a BOSU.

Sets: Three sets of 10 to 15 repetitions each leg.

3. Abdominals over Stability Ball with Medicine Ball

Functionality: To strengthen abdominals, core, and upper body.

Start by sitting on a stability ball holding a medicine ball in your hands. Walk your feet out from the ball and bring the medicine ball over your head. Begin the exercise by engaging your abdominals and raise the medicine ball over your head and up to almost a sitting position. Return to the start position and repeat. (See photos 16a and 16b.)

First Progression: Same as above, except start with your arms extended straight over your head for the entire exercise from start to finish.

Second progression: Same as above except start this exercise sitting on a BOSU.

Sets: Three sets of 15 to 20 repetitions.

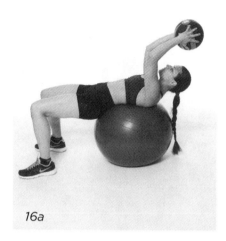

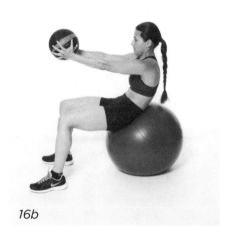

16a   16b

When we are in our racing season, we'll flip the switch again and move to a maintenance program, our in-season program, which will help us maintain solid function of our core and muscles. We'll take the number of exercises down to four exercises one day a week to coincide with our racing season.

In-Season Exercises

1. Superman on BOSU
2. Alternating Side Planks
3. One-Leg Hip Extensions on Floor
4. Opposite Arm and Leg Extension

1. Superman on BOSU

Functionality: To strengthen your back, shoulders, glutes, hamstrings, abdominals, and core.

Start by lying facedown with your hips centered on the BOSU, your legs straight and hip width apart, and your arms at your sides with palms facing down. Extend your shoulder blades back and down toward your spine. Inhale to prepare for the movement and then exhale as you extend your lower back, squeezing your glutes as you extend your torso up while rotating your thumbs toward the ceiling. Hold for 1 second in that position before returning to the start position.

First progression: Same as above, except raise your arms over your head and perform the movement without palms facing down. (See photos 17a and 17b.)

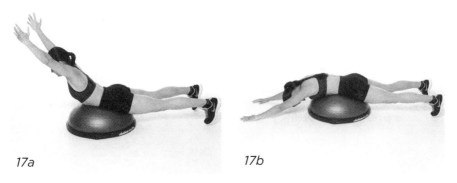

17a   17b

Second progression: Start by lying facedown, balanced on your midsection over the BOSU, with legs extended and arms overhead. Raise your legs and arms off the floor, find your balance, and then perform a swimming-type movement by fluttering your arms and legs for about 30 to 60 seconds.

Sets: Three sets of 15 repetitions.

2. Alternating Side Planks

Functionality: To strengthen your obliques, abdominals, core, shoulders and arms.

Start in a plank position with legs and arms straight, just beyond shoulder width apart. Shift your weight to one side and raise your opposite arm straight up toward the ceiling into a side plank position. Return controlled to a plank position and repeat on the opposite side. (See photos 18a and 18b.)

First progression: Begin by performing a push-up and then shift your weight to one side and raise your opposite arm straight up toward the ceiling into a side plank position. Return controlled to a plank position, and repeat the push-up and rotate to the opposite side. Split the desired number of repetitions between the sides.

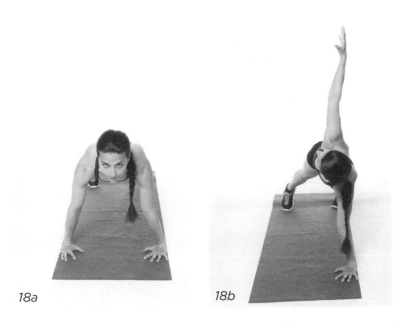

18a   *18b*

Sets: Three sets of 10 to 15 repetitions each side / first progression: three sets of 5 to 10 each side.

3. One-Leg Hip Extensions on Floor

Functionality: To strengthen your glutes, hamstrings, and quads.

Start by lying on your back on the floor with your knees bent and your arms out to the sides. Raise one leg straight out to the height of the opposite knee. Begin by extending your hips upward, forming a straight line from your

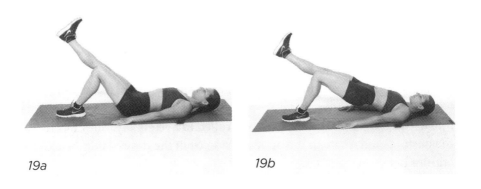

19a   *19b*

shoulder and with your thighs next to each other. Hold that position for 1 second and then return to the starting position on the floor. Repeat the desired number of repetitions before switching legs. (See photos 19a and 19b.)

First progression: same as above except start with one leg elevated on a step and perform the same movement.

Sets: Three sets of 15 repetitions each leg.

4. Opposite Arm and Leg Extension

Functionality: To strengthen your glutes and core.

Start by lying flat on your stomach with your arms above your head and thumbs pointing toward the ceiling. Raise one leg off the floor and simultaneously raise the opposite arm off the floor. Hold for at least 5 to 10 seconds before returning both your arm and leg back to the floor. Repeat this movement with the opposite leg and arm.

First progression: Same as above except start on your hands and knees with your hands directly under your shoulders and knees under your hips. Pull your belly button toward your spine as you engage your core and keep your back neutral. Extend one leg straight back and raise the opposite arm until they are in alignment with the body, holding for at least 5 to 10 seconds before returning to the starting position. Then repeat the movement with the opposite leg and arm. Keep alternating for the desired number of repetitions. (See photos 20a and 20b.)

Second progression: Same as first progression except in a plank position with legs and arms straight.

Sets: Three sets of 10 repetitions each side for 5- to 10-second hold on each side.

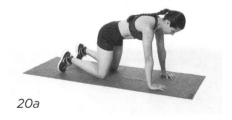
20a

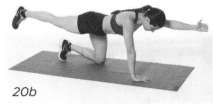
20b

These four in-season exercise sessions will help you to remain strong and healthy throughout the year and complete your overall training regimen.

To complement our functional core and strength training programs, we'll take you through a simple but effective warm-up and body preparation routine.

Warm-Up and Body-Preparation Routine

As we mentioned earlier, another important aspect of training and racing is preparing our bodies for activity. To do this, we want to raise our core body temperature and ready our joints, tendons, and muscles for the activity we are about to perform. After sitting for many hours or sleeping overnight, our bodies lose their elasticity. Often the spine and pelvis are not quite aligned and we can experience general stiffness.

To help remedy this, we'll start with some basic pre-movement exercises that you can use any time before a core and strength–training workout, or cardio workout, or even before a race, to open up your hips and realign your spine and pelvis to neutral.

The Simple Six offer a great way to wake up your body and ready you for an effective workout.

1. Pelvic Circles
Start in a standing position with your feet beyond shoulder width apart and hands on your waist. Begin by moving your hips in a counterclockwise circle

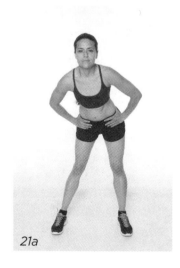
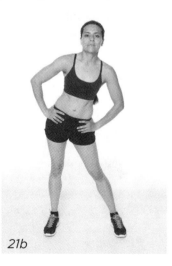

21a   21b

for 10 repetitions, feeling your pelvis and spine loosen. Then, move your hips in a clockwise circle for another 10 repetitions. (See photos 21a and 21b.)

2. Lunge Position Arm Reach

From the pelvic circles, starting in a standing position, raise both arms straight up over your head and lunge forward with your right leg. After you lunge forward, rotate your torso with arms raised to your left and then to your right. Return to the start position and repeat the lunge with your other leg. (See photos 22a and 22b.)

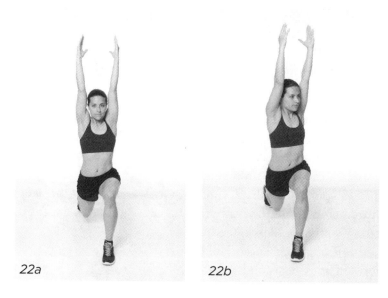

22a   *22b*

3. Back Stretch over Stability Ball

From a sitting position on the stability ball, walk your feet out from the ball while keeping your back in contact with the ball as you bring your shoulders and head back onto the ball. Then raise your arms out to the sides and extend backwards over the ball, again keeping your

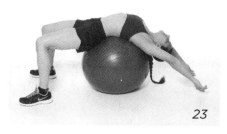

23

back and head in contact with the ball. Hold each stretch for about 20 to 30 seconds. (See photo 23.)

4. Side Stretch over Stability Ball

From the back stretch position, turn slightly onto your side while bringing your top arm over your head and holding on to the ball with your bottom arm. Let your hips and chest open up as you extend sideways over the ball. Hold the stretch for 30 seconds and then rotate to the opposite side, switching your arms' positions and holding that position for 30 seconds. (See photo 24.)

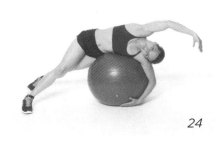

24

5. Hip Extensions

Lie down on the floor with your legs straight and arms at your side. Bend your knees and extend your hips up to form a straight line from your shoulders to your knees. Bring your hands together underneath your butt by pressing your shoulders into the floor and opening your chest. Hold that position for 30 seconds, then bring your hips back down to the floor and repeat for another 30-second hold. (See photo 25.)

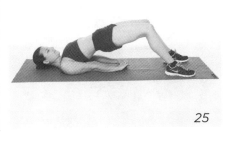

25

6. Press-Ups

From the hip extension, roll onto your stomach facedown with hands next to your shoulders and bent arms. Begin by pressing up with your arms, keeping your head in alignment with your spine. Extend to the point where you can keep your hips on the

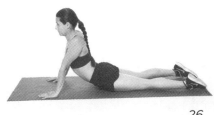

26

90

ground. Your glutes should be relaxed and allow your belly to fall to the floor. Hold and then return to starting position before continuing for a total of 10 repetitions. (See photo 26.)

This is a very simple routine that you can do in a matter of minutes, and it will have you feeling ready for a great workout!

Aside from preparing your body to work out, you also want to help your body recover from a workout. After a long workout, doing a repetitive-type movement like swimming, cycling, or running, your muscles tend to shorten and lose function. To help remedy this, we want to elongate the muscles to allow our spine and pelvis to realign and come back to neutral.

Flexibility and Stretching

We'll start with the big lower leg muscles and work our way through the entire body. Again, similar to our pre-movement exercises, these stretches can take as little 5 to 10 minutes or as long as 15 minutes depending on how much time you have and how much stretching you require.

1. Downward Dog Hamstring and Calf Stretch

Start in kneeling position with your legs and hands beyond hip and shoulder width apart. Lean forward with your hands over your head in a downward dog position, pushing your hips high and straightening your legs to create a straight line from your hands to your hips with your head down and arms straight. Hold the stretch for 20 to 30 seconds. To advance the stretch, go one toe of one foot and bring the other leg behind it. Then bring the calf to the floor to stretch it, and repeat with the other leg. (See photo 27.)

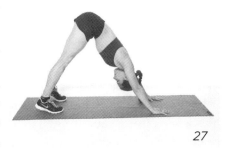

27

2. Psoas-to-Hip Flexor Stretch

From the downward dog position, stand up and take a big step forward to the wall or ground so your quadriceps is parallel to the ground and your back leg is slightly bent. Place your hands on your lead leg quadriceps, bring your chest

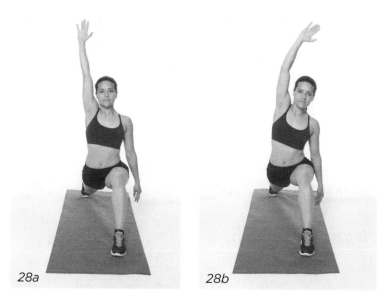

28a   28b

up and then raise the opposite arm straight up and hold that stretch for 20 seconds. Then bend your arm slightly over your head to stretch your hip flexor. Again, hold that stretch for 20 to 30 seconds and then return to the start position and repeat with the opposite leg and arm. (See photos 28a and 28b.)

3. Hamstring Stretch and Shoulder Stretch

Start in a standing position and cross one foot in front of the other while clasping your hands behind your back. Then, bend forward at your hips while raising your arms straight over your head. Hold that position for 20 seconds before returning to the start position. Then repeat by crossing the other foot and switching your handgrip and repeating the movement for another 20-second hold. (See photo 29.)

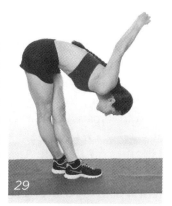

29

4. Quadriceps Stretch

Start in standing position, sideways to a wall or fence, grab your left foot behind you with your right hand, keeping your left knee next to your right knee. Hold that stretch for 20 to 30 seconds and then repeat on the other side with your left hand holding your right foot behind you. (See photo 30.)

5. Standing Piriformis Stretch

Again, standing sideways to a wall or fence, cross one leg over your knee and push your hips back close to a sitting position by bending the support leg. Hold this position for 20 to 30 seconds and then repeat with the opposite leg crossed over. (See photo 31.)

6. Standing Groin Stretch

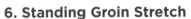

From a standing position, with your feet beyond shoulder width apart, push your hips and buttock back as you slide your hands down the front of your legs to your shins, eventually bending your knees and bringing your buttock toward the floor. Hold that stretch for 20 to 30 seconds. (See photo 32.)

7. Chest, Shoulder, and Neck Stretch

From a standing position with feet about shoulder width apart, place both hands behind your back and hold them together in an interlocking grip,

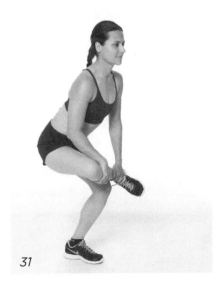

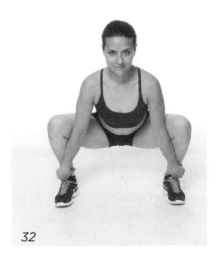

31

32

pulling your shoulder blades down and pulling your chest out while turning your head to the right and then to the left. Hold that position for 20 to 30 seconds. (See photo 33.)

We have seen great results with our athletes who use these functional strength and core sessions, pre-movement exercises, and warm-up exercises and hope you will give them a try too. And don't forget to work on your flexibility and stretching after workouts to keep you healthy and injury-free. They will give you a solid foundation of strength to draw upon and keep you injury-free as you go through the various training cycles of triathlon and embark on your journey to becoming or improving your triathlon performance.

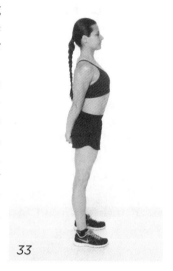

33

CHAPTER 8

The Crucial Training Principles and Training Cycles

To acquire knowledge one must study; but
to acquire wisdom, one must observe.

*—Marilyn vos Savant, author, lecturer, and
former Guinness Records "Highest IQ"*

Oh, good! You *are* reading this chapter. We were worried you might skip this one.

You see, one thing we have learned through many years of coaching is that most athletes are not interested in a lot of the science talk and lingo. Sure, a few are, and there are books that cover some of the very technical aspects of training in greater detail, but we know this is not what most athletes want.

Most athletes are busy people with careers, families, and other obligations, and what they want is a great plan and a clear path to accomplishing their goals. And just like our other books, that is exactly what we are providing here.

In fact, we have whittled it all down to four specific training concepts that we would like you to understand. Sure these concepts are all built right into the training plans in this book, but we have found that the athletes who do embrace these basic concepts are also the ones who are the most successful in the long run.

The four basic concepts and topics you can greatly benefit from are:

1. The Overload Principle
2. Training volume
3. Training cycles
4. Training races

Below we provide a concise explanation of each and we tell you exactly what you need to know to be most successful with the plans in this book.

The Overload Principle

The Overload Principle is the most fundamental concept of athletic training. The American Council on Exercise defines the Overload Principle as "One of the principles of human performance that states that beneficial adaptations occur in response to demands applied to the body at levels beyond a certain threshold (overload), but within the limits of tolerance and safety." In simple terms, our bodies either need to work harder or in a different way than they are used to working in order to improve.

If we regularly do the exact same volume of training, we will eventually hit a plateau and our fitness and performance will no longer improve. In fact, it will become stagnant and eventually probably even decline.

We need to introduce gradual "overloads" to our training volume in order to stimulate improvement. The overload needs to be just the right amount to stimulate the fitness improvements we want. The programs presented in this book are designed to do exactly that.

While the Overload Principle seems to make perfect sense, it is probably the single most violated principle we see among self-trained athletes. For example, we frequently see athletes who basically do the same limited number of workouts all of the time. The athletes are creatures of habit and they get stuck in their comfort zones. They like a workout and it makes them feel good, so why not do it three times a week for the remainder of eternity?

Well, of course, the Overload Principle tells us why. If you don't properly change the stimuli, then you do not promote fitness improvement and growth. Sure, for a while you see improvement, but then your fitness hits a plateau. Eventually, your fitness may even start to decline.

The other extreme is the athlete who makes radical changes in her workout from day to day. She does nothing or very little some days and she does far too much on other days. She quickly becomes injured. Her body cannot adapt to this "too little, too much" pattern and instead breaks down.

So keep these examples in mind and don't allow yourself to fall into these traps. The programs in this book are designed with this in mind. The workouts change and evolve over time, and they do so with the Overload Principle in mind.

Training Volume

The reason we want to briefly discuss training volume is simply because the majority of athletes do not actually know what it means. We are often surprised to find that most athletes equate training volume with duration. They think that the term "training volume" simply refers to the amount of time you train. Unfortunately, this mistake leads many self-trained athletes to performance stagnancy and injury.

Actually, volume is the combination of training duration, training frequency, and training intensity. The following equation is a great way to visualize this concept:

$$\text{Volume} = \text{Duration} \times \text{Frequency} \times \text{Intensity}$$

Our volume can increase as a result of increased training durations, but it can also increase as a result of higher training intensity, more frequent training sessions, or any combination of the three factors.

It is common to see athletes increase all three of these factors at the same time. They decide to "take their training up a notch" and begin training longer, harder, and more frequently . . . all at once. As we know from the Overload Principle described above, this can be a risky thing to do.

Many injuries in endurance sports are often blamed on "overtraining." What we usually find "overtraining" to actually mean is "too much, too soon." It's not simply that the athlete increased her durations too much, but she increased her frequency and intensity at the same time. She didn't give her body enough time to gradually adapt to these multiple changes in training volume factors, and her body broke down.

So, keep the components of training volume in mind, and don't allow yourself to fall into the "too much, too soon" trap. The programs in this book are designed with this in mind. The workouts are designed to properly coordinate training durations, intensities, and frequencies to maximize training results.

Training Cycles

As mentioned earlier, many athletes make the mistake of training pretty much the same way all of the time . . . no matter what time of the year it is, no matter which distance they are training for, and no matter what the timing and spacing of their races are. This results in ineffective training and performance stagnation. While an athlete may see improvement in the beginning, they eventually will plateau and then even start to decline. This is why we always want to train with proper training and racing cycles in mind.

In regard to our races, there are always three cycles occurring simultaneously:

1. The weekly cycle
2. The "A race" cycle
3. The annual training cycle

The weekly training cycle refers to the specific sessions we do each week and the days on which we do them. We do not do the exact same workout every day, but we do want to have a weekly pattern of the days on which we execute the eight key workouts referred to earlier. So for example, while we won't do the exact same long-run session every week, we will likely do our long-run session on the same day each week.

There are two big advantages for doing this. First, it's more efficient because it makes planning the rest of your life around your training much simpler. Secondly, and more important, it allows us to order our training sessions in the optimal way in which to maximize their training value. If training sessions are properly positioned throughout the week in relation to one another, we can increase their benefit and achieve truly synergistic training.

All of the training programs in this book are designed with the concept of weekly cycles in mind. The training sessions within each week are arranged in a pattern that maximizes their benefit.

The "A race" cycle is the training phase built around each A race. An A race is one that you consider to be one of your most important races of the year, and much or all of the year is focused on maximizing your performance in these races. Sure, you may have several other "B races" and "C races" too, but your A races are your primary focus. In general, most athletes do best with from one to four A races per year.

Any of the training programs in this book could possibly, although not necessarily, represent an A-race training cycle. Surely the programs for the

Half Iron-Distance (sixteen weeks plus) and the Full Iron-Distance (twenty to thirty weeks) do, but depending on your goals and focus, the training periods for Sprint and Standard Distance Races can be A-race training cycles as well.

Most A-race cycles, especially the longer ones, will include various training phases. First there's a phase to build an aerobic base, then a phase bringing in higher-intensity training, then a build to a peak level of training volume, and then a taper phase to have you rested, sharp, and race ready just when you need to be. As you will see in the training programs, each of these phases varies somewhat, depending on the race distance.

Finally, there is the annual training cycle. This refers to your entire year, which is going to be made up of perhaps several A-race cycles and likely even an off-season maintenance training phase (See Chapter 16). We have purposely designed this book in a way so that you can select from the various race-specific training programs in Chapters 10, 11, and 12, and the off-season maintenance program in Chapter 16, and put together your entire annual training cycle.

Training Races

Finally, we will touch on training races, which are clearly not "A races." These are the "other" races in your racing schedule. Some athletes pack their schedule with many of these other races and some don't have any at all. There are negatives with both extremes.

On the one hand, if you race too often, you may actually hurt your potential for achieving your goals in your A races. All of that racing tends to squeeze out the needed training sessions and it leaves the athlete run-down as opposed to built up. We often come across this extreme with athletes who like to race and don't really like to train that much. They often tell themselves, "I will race myself into shape," but this is a flawed approach and leads to inferior race preparation.

On the other hand, if you don't race enough, you tend to lose your "race sharpness." There is nothing like a race to practice and fine-tune your transition performance, your pre-race, race, and post-race fueling, hydration, and other racing routines, and to test out your race equipment, race clothing, and racing logistics. Athletes who rarely race tend to make mistakes in all of these key areas, and of course in triathlon, mistakes equate to lost time.

Racing prepares your body for the level of physical and mental intensity that is hard to re-create in training.

Optimally, there is a specific amount of racing that will contribute to your A-race performance. In each of the training programs in this book, we provide suggestions on what types of training races you should consider for each distance of A race and both when and how to build them into your training plan.

There we have it, the four key training concepts we need to embrace for success: the Overload Principle, training volume, training cycles, and training races.

Following is the seventh of seven motivating profiles of an inspiring female triathlete.

ATHLETE SUCCESS STORY:
KELLIE BROWN

Kellie Brown has been married for over fourteen years, she is a practicing veterinarian, and she has been competing in triathlon for over ten years. Over this time Kellie has raced in more than thirty events including virtually all distances short and long. While she enjoys all triathlon distances, Kellie likes long course distances like the Iron-Distance the most. Every year she has worked hard to hone her skills in the three disciplines and build her performances to the ranks of an elite-level-age-group triathlete. She has earned both overall victories at regional races and age-group podium finishes at national-class- and even world-class-level events.

Kellie's husband, Don, is also a competitive endurance athlete, so together they have become experts on how married couples can successfully train for and compete as athletes. As those of you who currently race along with your spouse know, there are pros and cons to having both of you pursing your athletic goals in the same sport. This is especially true if both individuals are competitive in nature and both want to excel. Of course, it adds to the experience if both individuals enjoy competing with each other and the competition can be positive and motivating.

According to Kellie, "When my husband first got into triathlon, I was a better athlete than he was. Now that he has a few seasons under his belt, he is faster and I'm a little jealous. But it motivates me to keep working hard and try to get faster and keep up! We don't mind a little healthy competition. Thankfully he is proud of my achievements and has always been incredibly supportive."

We have found this to be true for many of the married couples we have coached over the years. As long as you can be each other's biggest fan, then everything else can be worked through fairly easily.

Competing together has worked well for Kellie and her husband and we have heard this from other athletes and can include ourselves as well—it is a lot of fun to have your spouse in the race and know he or she is on the course, whether ahead or behind you. And although it does take some planning in terms of logistics, it is a great bonding experience.

Additional great tips from Kellie Brown:

- "Try to do some—but definitely not all—your training together. The sports where your abilities are the closest often work the best. But sharing a swim lane can work well even if your swim levels are not that close."
- "It's fine to race minor races together, but don't have the same A races. There is often too much stress around a big race, so it's best when the nonracing spouse can focus on supporting the racing spouse instead of being focused on his or her own race."

CHAPTER 9

Mastering Effective Heart Rate Training for Women

Your genetics load the gun,
the lifestyle pulls the trigger.

*—Mehmet Oz (aka Dr. Oz), cardiothoracic
surgeon, author, and television personality*

In this chapter we will explain what you need to know about our bodies'
energy systems; the importance of proper heart rate training; and how to
calculate your own unique heart rate zones to be used in the training programs in this book.

As we have said before, we will not go into a lot of scientific lingo like
they do in other books, because after having worked with hundreds and hundreds of athletes over many years, we know that is not what the vast majority
of athletes want. Most athletes want information and a great plan that they
can immediately put to work for them and see positive results. That is exactly
what we will present in this chapter: the basics of what you need to know and
how to make it work for you.

We will begin with a brief discussion about our bodies' energy systems
and what you need to know.

Aerobic versus Anaerobic

The body's two main energy systems are the following:

1. **Aerobic Energy System:** An energy system that utilizes oxygen
   and stored fat to power physical activity. This system can support
   activity for prolonged periods of time, as stored fat and oxygen are

available in almost endless supply. Even a very lean triathlete with a body-fat percentage in the single digits has enough stored fat to run several triathlons back-to-back.

2. **Anaerobic Energy System:** An energy system that utilizes glycogen (stored sugar) to power muscle activity. This system cannot support activity for long periods of time, as the body stores sugar in relatively small quantities.

While both of these energy systems work at the same time, the ratio of the two systems changes as the level of activity changes. The intensity of our training activity determines the ratio at which we are drawing from each system: The higher the intensity, the more anaerobic the activity; the lower the intensity, the more aerobic the activity.

Heart rate is an excellent indicator of where we are in the spectrum of aerobic and anaerobic ratios. At lower heart rates the mix is more aerobic. At higher heart rates the mix is more anaerobic. As our effort level and heart rate increase, the mix becomes more anaerobic.

For example, we race the shorter Sprint Distance Triathlon at a higher level of intensity than we do the much longer full Iron-Distance Triathlon. Therefore, the Sprint Distance Triathlon is a more anaerobic race than is the full Iron-Distance.

The important point to understand is that the benefit of an effective heart rate training program is that you are training at the proper intensity level at the right time, which serves to develop both your aerobic and anaerobic systems.

The "Train as You Feel" Myth

There is a fairly widely held misconception that you should always "train how you feel" and "go at your own pace." While there is some truth to this within certain boundaries, the reality is that how we feel is not usually the best indicator of the intensity level we should train at. Very often how we feel will put us at the wrong level of intensity at the wrong time, which leads to highly ineffective training. This is what we often refer to as "junk training."

In fact, what we have observed through our many years of training is that if an athlete trains how they feel, they tend to gravitate toward a fairly narrow range of intensities. Their "hard" days are a few heartbeats per minute higher and their "easy" days are a few heartbeats lower, but the vast majority of their training gravitates to the same narrow range of heart rates. Many refer to this narrow range as "the gray zone." While training in the gray zone may at first help a new athlete to improve her performance, before long she enters a period of performance stagnation, which can even lead to illness or injury.

If you are one of these gray zone trainers, don't despair. In fact, it is actually good news. It means that you are likely to have untapped athletic potential. The first step to releasing that potential is to begin training in the proper heart rate zones at the right time. A good heart rate–based training program is the key.

To have truly beneficial training for your event, there are specific intensity levels at which you should train to maximize the benefit of your training time. The reality is that for each race distance, a proper heart rate zone exists in which an athlete should train to maximize the benefit of her training time, as well as to avoid stagnation and even injury.

And the beauty of heart rate training is your ability to see your fitness gains in real terms. The fitter you get, the faster you will have to bike or run to stay at the same heart rate level. For example, for that hill you used to climb that made your heart rate soar into Z4 if you didn't slow down, you will now be able to take it at a slightly faster pace and keep your heart rate in Z2.

Calculating Heart Rate Zones for Women

The best way to determine your maximum heart rate (MHR) and heart rate training zones is to be formally tested. Many universities and sports fitness centers provide this type of testing for a reasonable cost.

If formal testing is not available, there are various popular formulas that can provide an estimate of your maximum heart rate. The most popular of all is the old "220 Minus Your Age" test. This test, for example, would estimate a forty-year-old man's MHR to be about 180 beats per minute (BPM) as follows:

MHR using "220 – Your Age" for a 40-year-old man:
220 – 40 = 180 BPM

However, the "220 Minus Your Age" formula was based on males and not females. Due to generally slightly higher MHR for women compared to men, the above formula is often adjusted slightly to "226 Minus Your Age" for women. Based on this version of the formula, a forty-year-old woman's MHR would be estimated as follows:

MHR using "226 – Your Age" for a 40-year-old woman:
226 – 40 = 186

There are many other popular tests for estimating your MHR as well. For example, fitness writer Jenny Sugar suggests the following formula, developed at Northwestern Medicine in Chicago, for estimating a woman's maximum heart rate:

MHR = 206 – (88% of Your Age).

But the important point is that these tests are only estimates and cannot be completely relied upon. While these tests can provide a starting point, we suggest using simple field tests to double-check your MHR.

The first simple field test is to run a 5K race or time trial at a 100 percent effort and to record your MHR during the effort. This is very likely your MHR for running.

Once you have determined your maximum heart rate, we can use it to determine the four training zones for use with the training plans presented in this book:

Zone 4: 90% to 95% of MHR (anaerobic training)

Zone 3: 86% to 89% of MHR (middle zone)

Zone 2: 75% to 85% of MHR (higher-end aerobic training)

Zone 1: 65% to 74% of MHR (lower-end aerobic training)

As an example, for a forty-year-old female athlete with an estimated 186 MHR, her heart rate zones for running would be as follows:

Running Heart Rate Zones

Z4: 90% to 95% of 186 MHR = 167 to 177 beats per minute (BPM)

Z3: 86% to 89% of 186 MHR = 159 to 166 BPM

Z2: 75% to 85% of 186 MHR = 139 to 158 BPM

Z1: 65% to 74% of 186 MHR = 121 to 138 BPM

Because cycling stresses our bodies in different ways than running (e.g., sitting vs. standing and more balanced vs. less balanced), our heart rates for cycling are usually about 5 percent lower than our running heart rate zones. In other words, when cycling we obtain the equivalent training effect at a heart rate about 5 percent lower than when running.

In the following table we apply 95 percent (a 5 percent decrease to the same forty-year-old athlete's running heart rate zones to estimate her heart rate zones for training on the bike:

RUNNING ZONES	CYCLING ZONES (95% OF RUN ZONES)
Z4 = 167 to 177 BPM	Z4 = 159 to 168 BPM
Z3 = 159 to 166 BPM	Z3 = 151 to 158 BPM
Z2 = 139 to 158 BPM	Z2 = 132 to 150 BPM
Z1 = 121 to 138 BPM	Z1 = 115 to 131 BPM

While this 95 percent guideline provides a pretty close estimate for the majority of athletes, we usually encourage our coached athletes to do another simple field test. To determine your MHR for the bike, we suggest a 100-percent-effort 15-minute cycling time trial (do this on a flat, safe course with no traffic) with a heart rate monitor and confirm your maximum heart rate for the bike. This field test is usually a very good indication of your maximum cycling heart rate. If your field test results differ, adjust your heart rate zones accordingly.

To summarize, the best approach is to have formal testing. But if formal testing is not possible, we suggest you use the "226 Minus Your Age" estimate (and/or the alternative method developed at Northwestern Medicine presented above) as a starting point and then double-check your results with both the 100-percent-effort 5K run and 100-percent-effort 15-minute cycling time trial. This will provide you with good heart rate zones to work with for training programs in this book.

Special Women-Specific Heart Rate Issues

Below are three special issues affecting heart rates that are unique to women:

1. Menstrual cycle

In the old days it was generally believed that women should not participate in athletics during their menstrual cycle, but today it is generally accepted that women can train and even race while menstruating. In fact, having coached hundreds of women over the years, we know firsthand that many women compete very successfully during the menstrual cycle. What's more, women who exercise regularly tend to experience shorter and less extreme menstrual cycles. This is yet another of the many advantages to being an endurance athlete.

We discuss menstrual cycles in more detail in Chapter 15, but our focus in this chapter is the impact of menstrual cycles on heart rate levels. Many women find that due to fluctuating hormone levels at the start of their menstrual cycles, they experience slightly elevated heart rates. While this does not mean you shouldn't train or race, it may mean that your performance may be impacted by the higher heart rates. Because of this and some of the other issues concerning menstrual cycles, most professional triathletes and more serious amateur athletes try to time their race dates and menstrual cycles accordingly so as not to intersect. If planned out several months in advance, most women can fairly easily accomplish this.

2. Heat and humidity

Women have a tendency to be able to tolerate heat and humidity better than their male counterparts simply due to their smaller size. As we exercise, we produce heat, and our ability to get rid of that heat as quickly as possible will help us to perform better. A woman's relative smaller size to skin surface creates a better ability to reduce heat. That is not to say this does not apply to a smaller male athlete as well. The important point, however, is that because of this, women's heart rates tend to be less affected in general by heat and humidity than most men.

3. Athletic ability

One thing we have found in coaching women and some men is that many do not have the ability to push themselves in training or even a race situation to anywhere near their maximum heart rate. This may be due to their relative athletic ability or simply strength and fitness. Or they may not be willing to stress their bodies or push themselves in a way in which they "have to suffer." Or they may feel they will injure themselves. This is understandable, however, it can make it difficult to predict their true maximum heart rate and resulting proper heart rate zones.

An IronFit Moment

Lactate Threshold

Many athletes hear the term "lactate threshold," but few really understand what it is and what it means in the context of effective training. "Lactate threshold" is the heart rate level at which lactate begins to accumulate at a faster rate in the muscles than the body can clear.

Lactate is produced in our bodies when performing physical activity. The accumulation of lactate has a negative impact on the muscles' ability to perform. Lactate threshold is not a constant. It changes relatively quickly for several reasons including changes in your fitness level. Daily variations of up to several heart beats per minute are common.

Another way to look at lactate threshold is that it is approximately the heart rate a well-trained athlete can maintain for about one hour at 100 percent effort. This can be helpful to know as it implies that for any distance you race that takes you less than one hour, you should be mostly at a heart rate higher than your lactate threshold. For any distance that takes you longer than one hour to complete, you should be mostly at a heart rate under your lactate threshold.

CHAPTER 10

Training Programs for Sprint and Standard Distance Triathlons

This chapter includes three detailed Eight-Week Sprint Distance (approximately a 0.5-mile swim, 15-mile bike, and 3-mile run) and Standard Distance (1.5-km swim, 40-km bike, and 10-km run) training programs. Each program is based on the number of hours an athlete has available to train. The Competitive Program includes about twelve peak weekly hours; the Intermediate Program includes about nine peak weekly hours; and the Just-Finish Program has about six peak weekly hours.

Each program tells the reader exactly what to do each and every day throughout the eight-week period. There are none of the complicated formulas or overly general workout descriptions often found in other training books. Having worked with hundreds of female athletes for many years, we know that this is not what you want. Athletes want clear direction on exactly what they need to do and when. This is exactly what this chapter provides. The programs are designed to be efficient, productive, and enjoyable.

Following is a summary comparison of the three eight-week programs:

TRAINING PROGRAM	AVERAGE HOURS/WEEK	PEAK HOURS/WEEK	TOTAL HOURS (APPROX.)
Competitive	10	12	80
Intermediate	7.5	9	60
Just-Finish	5	6	40

Consider the time management techniques presented in Chapter 2 and in the athlete profiles throughout this book, and conservatively estimate your weekly training time availability. Once you have completed this analysis, simply select the program that best fits you, your goals, your experience level, and your available training time.

Abbreviations for Training Programs

Following is an explanation of the abbreviations used in each of the training programs in this book:

Z1	Heart rate zone one (heart rate zones are explained in Chapter 9)
30 min.	Thirty minutes
1:15 hr.	One hour and fifteen minutes
100+RPM	Pedal bike at a cadence of 100 or more pedal revolutions per minute.
Trans	Transition sessions are a combined bike/run session, where we transition from one sport to the other in 5 minutes or less (transition sessions are discussed in Chapter 6).
QC	Quickly change from cycling gear to running gear within 5 minutes.
Z1 to Z2	Train at a heart rate anywhere within zone one and zone two (heart rate zones are discussed in Chapter 9).
30 min. Z2 (at 20 min., insert 5-min. Z4)	Begin the 30-minute session in your Z2 heart rate. At 20 minutes into the session, increase your heart rate to Z4 (by increasing your effort level) for 5 minutes. At the completion of the 5 minutes, return to Z2 for the remaining 5 minutes of the session.
PU	Pickups are temporary increases in effort by about 10% to 15%.
Spin	Easy recovery cycling in an easier gear.
Jog	Easy recovery running at a slower pace.

Sample bike training session: 45 min. Z2 (at 10 min., insert 5 x 4 min. Z4 @ 2 min. spin)

Begin your 45-minute bike session at a pace that will maintain a Z2 heart rate. At 10 minutes into the session, increase your heart rate to Z4 (by increasing your effort level) for 4 minutes and then decrease gearing for an easy 2-minute spin. Repeat this sequence five times. After completing five sequences return to a Z2 heart rate for the remainder of the 45-minute bike.

Sample run training session: 45 min. Z2 (at 10 min., insert 4 x 6 min. Z4 @ 3 min. jog)

> Begin your 45-minute run at a pace that will maintain a Z2 heart rate. At 10 minutes into the run, increase your effort enough to maintain a Z4 heart rate for a period of 6 minutes. After the 6 minutes slow down to an easy 3-minute jog, bringing your heart rate back down to Z1 or Z2. Repeat this sequence four times. After completing four sequences, return to a Z2 heart rate for the remainder of the run.

WU	Easy warm-up
CD	Easy cool-down
DR	Swim drills (swim drills are presented in Chapter 14.)

Notes to Swim Sessions in Training Programs

Perceived Effort: It is suggested you use the following perceived effort levels with the swim sessions:

- Warm-up, drills (see Chapter 14 for swim drills), and cool-down should be at a perceived effort of about 65% to 75%.
- Main swim sets should be at a perceived effort of about 80% to 85%.
- Main swim sets indicated as "fast" should be at a perceived effort of about 90% to 95%.

Here is an example of how to read a swim workout, with an explanation of the following swim session:

> 300 wu, 6x50 drills @ 10 sec., 10 x 100 @ 15 sec., 5 x 200 @ 20 sec., 6x50 drills @ 10 sec., 200cd

1. Start by swimming any easy 300 yards/meters (65% to 75% perceived effort).
2. Select one or more drills from Chapter 14 and swim it/them for 50 yards/meters. Rest for 10 seconds at the wall after completing the 50-yard/meter drill and then repeat this entire sequence for a

total of six times through, each time swimming 50 yards/meters of the drill and each time taking a 10-second rest after it (65% to 75% perceived effort).

3. Swim 100 yards/meters and stop at the wall for a 15-second rest. Repeat this entire sequence 10 times through (80% to 85% perceived effort).

4. Swim 200 yards/meters and stop at the wall for a 20-second rest. Repeat this entire sequence for a total of five times through (80% to 85% perceived effort).

5. Select one or more drills from Chapter 14 and swim it for 50 yards/meters. Rest for 10 seconds at the wall after completing the 50-yard/meter drill and then repeat this entire sequence for a total of six times through, each time swimming 50 yards/meters of the drill and each time taking a 10-second rest after it (65% to 75% perceived effort).

6. Finish by swimming an easy 200 yards/meters (65% to 75% perceived effort).

Swim Sessions

The following numbered swim sessions are to be used with the training programs in Chapters 10, 11, 12, and 16. Swim sessions 1 through 24 are all about 3,000 yards/meters; sessions 25 through 44 are all about 2,000 yards/meters; and swim sessions 45 through 60 are all about 2,500 yards/meters.

3,000-Yard/Meter Swim Sessions

1. 300 wu, 6 x 50 drills @ 10 sec., 7 x 50 @ 10 sec., 3 x 100 @ 20 sec., 3 x 200 @ 30 sec., 3 x 100 @ 20 sec., 7 x 50 @ 10 sec., 6 x 50 drills @ 10 sec., 200 cd

2. 300 wu, 6 x 50 drills @ 10 sec., 4 x (125 @ 10sec., 150 @ 15 sec., 200 @ 20 sec.), 6 x 50 drills @ 10 sec., 200 cd

3. 300 wu, 8 x 50 drills @ 10 sec., 7 x (25 @ 5 sec., 50 @ 10 sec., 75 @ 10 sec., 100 @ 20 sec.), 7 x 50 drills @ 10 sec., 200 cd

4. 300 wu, 6 x 50 drills @ 10 sec., 1 x 500 Pull @ 30 sec., 2 x 250 @ 20 sec., 4 x 125 @ 15 sec., 4 x 100 @ 10 sec., 6 x 50 drills @ 10 sec., 200 cd

5. 300 wu, 7 x 50 drills @ 10 sec., 3 x (100 @ 15 sec., 150 @ 20 sec., 100 @ 15 sec., 250 @ 30 sec.), 7 x 50 drills @ 10 sec., 200 cd

6. 300 wu, 7 x 50 drills @ 10 sec., 8 x 25 @ 5 sec., 4 x 50 @ 10 sec., 4 x 100 @ 15 sec., 3 x 200 Pull @ 20 sec., 1 x 400 @ 30 sec., 7 x 50 drills @ 10 sec., 200 cd

7. 300 wu, 7 x 50 drills @ 10 sec., 3 x (4 x 100 @ 10 sec., 1 x 200 @ 20 sec.), 7 x 50 drills @ 10 sec., 200 cd

8. 300 wu, 7 x 50 drills @ 10 sec., 6 x 175 @ 20 sec., 6 x 125 @ 10 sec., 7 x 50 drills @ 10 sec., 200 cd

9. 300 wu, 6 x 50 drills @ 10 sec., 500 Pull @ 35 sec., 400 @ 30 sec., 300 Pull @ 25 sec., 200 @ 20 sec., 5 x 100 @ 15 sec., 6 x 50 drills @ 10 sec., 200 cd

10. 300 wu, 5 x 50 drills @ 10 sec., 4 x (50 @ 5 sec., 100 @ 10 sec., 150 @ 15sec., 200 @ 20 sec.), 5 x 50 drills @ 10 sec., 200 cd

11. 300 wu, 7 x 50 drills @ 10 sec., 3 x (75 @ 10 sec., 125 @ 15 sec., 175 @ 20 sec., 225 @ 25 sec.), 7 x 50 drills @ 10 sec., 200 cd

12. 300 wu, 7 x 50 drills @ 10 sec., 6 x 25 @ 5 sec., 6 x 75 @ 10 sec., 4 x 150 @ 15 sec., 6 x 75 @ 10 sec., 6 x 25 @ 5 sec., 7 x 50 drills @ 10 sec., 200 cd

13. 300 wu, 7 x 50 drills @ 10 sec., 4 x 200 Pull @ 20 sec., 4 x 150 @ 15 sec., 4 x 100 @ 10 sec., 7 x 50 drills @ 10 sec., 200 cd

14. 300 wu, 6 x 50 drills @ 10 sec., 3 x (4 x 75 @ 10 sec., 1 x 350 @ 30 sec.), 5 x 50 drills @ 10 sec., 200 cd

15. 300 wu, 6 x 50 drills @ 10 sec., 5 x 100 @ 10 sec., 6 x 150 @ 15 sec., 5 x 100 @ 10 sec., 6 x 50 drills @ 10 sec., 200 cd

16. 300 wu, 4 x 50 drills @ 10 sec., 3 x (1 x 400 Pull @ 30 sec., 3 x 100 @ 10 sec.), 4 x 50 drills @ 10 sec., 200 cd

17. 300 wu, 4 x 50 drills @ 10 sec., 3 x 100 @ 10 sec., 3 x 150 @ 15 sec., 3 x 200 @ 20 sec., 3 x 250 @ 25 sec., 4 x 50 drills @ 10 sec., 200 cd

18. 300 wu, 6 x 50 drills @ 10 sec., 4 x 75 @ 10 sec., 4 x 125 @ 15 sec., 1 x 300 @ 20 sec., 4 x 125 @ 15 sec., 4 x 75 @ 10 sec., 6 x 50 drills @ 10 sec., 200 cd

19. 300 wu, 5 x 50 drills @ 10 sec., 200 @ 20 sec., 300 @ 25 sec., 400 Pull @ 30 sec., 500 @ 35 sec., 600 Pull @ 40 sec., 5 x 50 drills @ 10 sec., 200 cd

20. 300 wu, 6 x 50 drills @ 10 sec., 12 x 25 @ 5 sec., 8 x 50 @ 10 sec., 5 x 100 @ 15 sec., 8 x 50 @ 10 sec., 12 x 25 @ 5 sec., 6 x 50 drills @ 10 sec., 200 cd

21. 300 wu, 4 x 50 drills @ 10 sec., 3 x (75 @ 10 sec., 125 @ 15 sec., 225 @ 20 sec., 275 @ 25 sec.), 4 x 50 drills @ 10 sec., 200 cd

22. 300 wu, 7 x 50 drills @ 10 sec., 8 x 75 @ 10 sec., 3 x 200 Pull @ 20 sec., 8 x 75 @ 10 sec., 7 x 50 drills @ 10 sec., 200 cd

23. 300 wu, 7 x 50 drills @ 10 sec., 50 @ 5 sec., 100 @ 10 sec., 150 @ 15 sec., 200 @ 20 sec., 250 @ 25 sec., 300 Pull @ 30 sec., 250 @ 25 sec., 200 @ 20 sec., 150 @ 15 sec., 100 @ 10 sec., 50 @ 5 sec., 7 x 50 drills @ 10 sec., 200 cd

24. 300 wu, 7 x 50 drills @ 10 sec., 6 x 200 @ 20 sec., 6 x 100 @ 15 sec., 7 x 50 drills @ 10 sec., 200 cd

2,000 Yards/Meters Swim Sessions

25. 200 wu, 5 x 50 drills @ 10 sec., 3 x 50 @ 10 sec., 2 x 100 @ 20 sec., 2 x 150 @ 30 sec., 3 x 100 @ 20 sec., 3 x 50 @ 10 sec., 5 x 50 drills @ 10 sec., 200 cd

26. 200 wu, 6 x 50 drills @ 10 sec., 4 x (100 @ 15 sec., 150 @ 20 sec.), 6 x 50 drills @ 10 sec., 200 cd

27. 200 wu, 6 x 50 drills @ 10 sec., 4 x (25 @ 5 sec., 50 @ 5 sec., 75 @ 10 sec., 100 @ 15 sec.), 6 x 50 drills @ 10 sec., 200 cd

28. 200 wu, 6 x 50 drills @ 10 sec., 2 x 250 Pull @ 30 sec., 4 x 125 @ 15 sec., 6 x 50 drills @ 10 sec., 200 cd

29. 200 wu, 6 x 50 drills @ 10 sec., 3 x (100 @ 15 sec., 250 @ 30 sec.), 6 x 50 drills @ 10 sec., 200 cd

30. 200 wu, 6 x 50 drills @ 10 sec., 8 x 25 @ 5 sec., 4 x 50 @ 10 sec., 2 x 100 @ 15 sec., 2 x 200 @ 20 sec., 6 x 50 drills @ 10 sec., 200 cd

31. 200 wu, 6 x 50 drills @ 10 sec., 3 x (150 @ 15 sec., 200 Pull @ 20 sec.), 6 x 50 drills @ 10 sec., 200 cd

32. 200 wu, 7 x 50 drills @ 10 sec., 3 x 175 @ 20 sec., 3 x 125 @ 10 sec., 7 x 50 drills @ 10 sec., 200 cd

33. 200 wu, 6 x 50 drills @ 10 sec., 400 @ 30 sec., 300 Pull @ 25 sec., 200 @ 20 sec., 100 @ 15 sec., 6 x 50 drills @ 10 sec., 200 cd

34. 200 wu, 6 x 50 drills @ 10 sec., 2 x (50 @ 5 sec., 100 @ 10 sec., 150 @ 15 sec., 200 @ 20 sec.), 6 x 50 drills @ 10 sec., 200 cd

35. 200 wu, 6 x 50 drills @ 10 sec., 3 x (125 @ 15 sec., 225 @ 25 sec.), 6 x 50 drills @ 10 sec., 200 cd

36. 200 wu, 6 x 50 drills @ 10 sec., 4 x 25 @ 5 sec., 2 x 75 @ 10 sec., 4 x 125 @ 15 sec., 2 x 75 @ 10 sec., 4 x 25 @ 5 sec., 6 x 50 drills @ 10 sec., 200 cd

37. 200 wu, 6 x 50 drills @ 10 sec., 4 x 150 @ 15 sec., 4 x 100 @ 10 sec., 6 x 50 drills @ 10 sec., 200 cd

38. 200 wu, 6 x 50 drills @ 10 sec., 4 x 250 @ 30 sec., 6 x 50 drills @ 10 sec., 200 cd

39. 200 wu, 7 x 50 drills @ 10 sec., 3 x (25 fast @ 15 sec., 125 @ 15 sec.), 3 x (50 fast @ 15, 100 @ 15), 7 x 50 drills @ 10 sec., 200 cd

40. 200 wu, 6 x 50 drills @ 10 sec., 1 x (3 x 200 @ 30 sec., 4 x 100 @ 15 sec., 6 x 50 drills @ 10 sec., 200 cd

41. 200 wu, 6 x 50 drills @ 10 sec., 3 x (25 @ 5 sec., 75 @ 10 sec., 100 @ 15 sec., 150 @ 20 sec.), 5 x 50 drills @ 10 sec., 200 cd

42. 200 wu, 7 x 50 drills @ 10 sec., 50 fast @ 10 sec., 100 pull @ 15 sec., 50 fast @ 10 sec., 150 pull @ 20 sec., 50 fast @ 10 sec., 200 pull @ 20 sec., 50 fast @ 10 sec., 250 pull @ 25 sec., 7 x 50 drills @ 10 sec., 200 cd

43. 200 wu, 6 x 50 drills @ 10 sec., 4 x 25 @ 10 sec., 4 x 50 @ 15 sec., 4 x 75 @ 15 sec., 4 x 100 fast @ 20 sec., 6 x 50 drills @ 10 sec., 200 cd

44. 200 wu, 6 x 50 drills @ 10 sec., 4 x (100 fast @ 15 sec., 150 pull @ 15 sec.), 6 x 50 drills @ 10 sec., 200 cd

2,500-Yard/Meter Swim Sessions

45. 200 wu, 6 x 50 drills @ 10 sec., 6 x 25 @ 5 sec., 2 x 50 @ 10 sec., 2 x 75 @ 10 sec., 2 x 100 @ 15 sec., 2 x 125 @ 15 sec.; 2 x 150 @ 15 sec., 2 x 175 @ 20 sec., 6 x 50 drills @ 10 sec., 200 cd

46. 200 wu, 7 x 50 drills @ 10 sec., 4 x (150 @ 15 sec., 200 Pull @ 20 sec.), 7 x 50 drills @ 10 sec., 200 cd

47. 200 wu, 6 x 50 drills @ 10 sec., 5 x 175 @ 20 sec., 5 x 125 @ 10 sec., 6 x 50 drills @ 10 sec., 200 cd

48. 200 wu, 6 x 50 drills @ 10 sec., 500 Pull @ 35 sec., 400 @ 30 sec., 300 Pull @ 25 sec., 200 @ 20 sec., 100 @ 15 sec., 6 x 50 drills @ 10 sec., 200 cd

49. 200 wu, 6 x 50 drills @ 10 sec., 3 x (50 @ 5 sec., 100 @ 10 sec., 150 @ 15 sec., 200 @ 20 sec.), 6 x 50 drills @ 10 sec., 200 cd

50. 200 wu, 7 x 50 drills @ 10 sec., 4 x (125 @ 15 sec., 225 @ 20 sec.), 7 x 50 drills @ 10 sec., 200 cd

51. 200 wu, 7 x 50 drills @ 10 sec., 4 x 25 @ 5 sec., 4 x 75 @ 10 sec., 4 x 150 @ 15 sec., 4 x 75 @ 10 sec., 4 x 25 @ 5 sec., 7 x 50 drills @ 10 sec., 200 cd

52. 200 wu, 6 x 50 drills @ 10 sec., 6 x 150 @ 15 sec., 6 x 100 @ 10 sec., 6 x 50 drills @ 10 sec., 200 cd

53. 200 wu, 6 x 50 drills @ 10 sec., 6 x 250 @ 30 sec., 6 x 50 drills @ 10 sec., 200 cd

54. 200 wu, 7 x 50 drills @ 10 sec., 4 x 100 @ 10 sec., 3 x 200 @ 15 sec., 4 x 100 @ 10 sec., 7 x 50 drills @ 10 sec., 200 cd

55. 200 wu, 6 x 50 drills @ 10 sec., 2 x 250 @ 20 sec., 1 x 500 Pull @ 30 sec., 2 x 250 @ 20 sec., 6 x 50 drills @ 10 sec., 200 cd

56. 200 wu, 6 x 50 drills @ 10 sec., 3 x (100 @ 10 sec., 150 @ 15 sec., 250 Pull @ 20 sec.), 6 x 50 drills @ 10 sec., 200 cd

57. 200 wu, 6 x 50 drill @ 10 sec., 6 x (25 @ 5 sec., 50 @ 10 sec., 75 @ 10 sec., 100 @ 20 sec.), 6 x 50 drills @ 10 sec., 200 cd

58. 200 wu, 6 x 50 drills @ 10 sec., 1 x 500 @ 30 sec., 2 x 250 @ 20 sec., 4 x 125 @ 15 sec., 6 x 50 drills @ 10 sec., 200 cd

59. 200 wu, 6 x 50 drills @ 10 sec., 3 x (100 @ 15 sec., 2 x 150 @ 20 sec., 100 @ 15 sec.), 6 x 50 drills @ 10 sec., 200 cd

60. 200 wu, 4 x 50 drills @ 10 sec., 8 x 25 @ 5 sec., 4 x 50 @ 10 sec., 4 x 100 @ 15 sec., 3 x 200 Pull @ 20 sec., 1 x 400 @ 30 sec., 4 x 50 drills @ 10 sec., 200 cd

Following are our three eight-week training programs and full explanations of each, starting with the Eight-Week Competitive Program:

Competitive Training Program for Sprint and Standard Distance Triathlons

The Competitive Program is for the experienced athlete who wants to maximize her potential and has available time to train for an average of about ten hours a week, with several peak weeks of about twelve hours. The total combined training time over the eight-week period is approximately eighty hours so we like to refer to this as the "eighty-hour plan."

If you are already in your racing season and in good form, you can begin the program immediately after your last race. The first week is fully aerobic, which will help to complete your recovery and firm up your aerobic base. Then in the second week we will include Easy Pickups on both the cycling and running sides to prepare us to transition into our higher-intensity sessions.

From there, our higher-intensity sessions and duration will build and become more challenging. We start at about nine hours of training in the first week and then gradually build by about one hour per week to about twelve hours in the fourth week. This amount assumes two swims of about one hour each per week, but this program also includes an optional third swim, which adds another hour to these totals. If swimming is your weakest of the three sports, it will be very helpful to include the third swim if possible.

Our quantity of Z4 training will gradually build and peak in week six at just over 100 minutes combined. Weeks three through six will each have four sessions that will include Z4 work, including two bike sessions and two run sessions. With seven bike and/or run sessions per week during this period, this means that more than half of the sessions (57%) will include Z4 higher-intensity training.

Our longest sessions in the eight weeks will be three three-hour transition sessions in weeks four, five, and six. Our longest runs of the eight weeks will be two two-hour sessions in weeks four and six of the program.

With nine days to go before our race, we will transition into our crisp taper phase to have us rested, sharp, and race-ready. Our durations will gradually decrease and our intensities will be no higher than Z2 during these last nine days. At this point the hay is in the barn and it is time to taper smart and become physically and mentally energized.

If you are not coming off a race or you have not already built up to or close to nine hours of training per week before starting the Competitive Program, it is suggested that you do. Depending on your starting point, complete four to eight weeks of moderate aerobic exercise to be properly prepared to begin the program. If you are starting from scratch, we suggest you start with two easy weekly swims of about 30 minutes, three easy bike sessions of about 30 to 45 minutes, and three easy run sessions of 30 to 45 minutes. Then, over the four- to eight-week period, make gradual increases each week until you are comfortably up to or close to the nine-hour level. Once there, you are ready to begin with the first week of the eight-week program.

Competitive Program
The following chart details the Eight-Week Competitive Program:

COMPETITIVE PROGRAM — SPRINT AND STANDARD DISTANCE TRIATHLONS

WEEK 1	SWIM	BIKE	RUN
M	#1—Opt.	Rest day/slide day	Rest day/slide day
T	Off	Off	45 min. Z2
W	#2	Trans: 45 min. Z2 (QC)	15 min. Z2
R	Off	45 min. Z2	Off
F	#3	Off	45 min. Z2
S	Off	Trans: 1:30 hr. Z2 (QC)	15 min. Z2
S	Off	30 min. Z1 (100+ rpm)	1:30 hr. Z1 to Z2
Totals: 9:00+ hr.	2:00+ hr.	3:30 hr.	3:30 hr.

WEEK 2	SWIM	BIKE	RUN
M	#4—Opt.	Rest day/slide day	Rest day/slide day
T	Off	Off	45 min. Z2 (at 10 min., insert 5 x 1 min. PU @ 1 min. jog)
W	#5	Trans: 45 min. Z2 (QC)	15 min. Z2
R	Off	60 min. Z2 (at 10 min., insert 5 x 1 min. PU @ 1 min. spin)	Off
F	#6	Off	60 min. Z2 (at 45 min., insert 5 min. Z4)
S	Off	Trans: 1:45 hr. Z2 (at 1:30, insert 10 min. Z4) (QC)	30 min. Z2
S	Off	30 min. Z1 (100+ rpm)	1:30 hr. Z1 to Z2
Totals: 10:00+ hr.	2:00+ hr.	4:00 hr.	4:00 hr.
WEEK 3	SWIM	BIKE	RUN
M	#7—Opt.	Rest day/slide day	Rest day/slide day
T	Off	Off	60 min. Z2 (at 10 min., insert 8 x 2 min. Z4 @ 1 min. jog)
W	#8	Trans: 45 min. Z2 (QC)	15 min. Z2
R	Off	60 min. Z2 (at 10 min., insert 5 x 4 min. Z4@ 2 min. spin; then 5 x 2 min. Z4@ 1 min. spin)	Off
F	#9	Off	60 min. Z2 (at 45 min., insert 10 min. Z4)
S	Off	Trans: 1:45 hr. Z2 (at 1:25, insert 15 min. Z4) (QC)	45 min. Z2
S	Off	60 min. Z1 (100+ rpm)	1:30 hr. Z1 to Z2
Totals: 11:00+ hr.	2:00+ hr.	4:30 hr.	4:30 hr.

COMPETITIVE PROGRAM — SPRINT AND STANDARD DISTANCE TRIATHLONS

WEEK 4	SWIM	BIKE	RUN
M	#10—Opt.	Rest day/slide day	Rest day/slide day
T	Off	Off	60 min. Z2 (at 10 min., insert 7 x 3 min. Z4 @ 1.5 min. jog)
W	#11	Trans: 45 min. Z2 (QC)	15 min. Z2
R	Off	60 min. Z2 (at 10 min., insert 10 x 3 min. Z4 Hill Repeats @ spin back down)	Off
F	#12	Off	60 min. Z2 (at 40 min., insert 15 min. Z4)
S	Off	Trans: 2:15 hr. Z2 (at 1:50, insert 20 min. Z4) (QC)	45 min. Z2
S	Off	60 min. Z1 (100+ rpm)	2:00 hr. Z1 to Z2
Totals: 12:00+ hr.	2:00+ hr.	5:00 hr.	5:00 hr.

WEEK 5	SWIM	BIKE	RUN
M	#13—Opt.	Rest day/slide day	Rest day/slide day
T	Off	Off	60 min. Z2 (at 10 min., insert 6 x 4.5 min. Z4 @ 2 min. jog)
W	#14	Trans: 45 min. Z2 (QC)	15 min. Z2
R	Off	60 min. Z2 (at 10 min., insert 2 x 5 min. Z4 @ 3 min. spin; then 5 x 4 min. Z4 @ 2 min. spin)	Off
F	#15	Off	60 min. Z2 (at 15 min., insert 15 min. Z4)
S	Off	Trans: 2:15 hr. Z2 (at 1:45, insert 25 min. Z4) (QC)	45 min. Z2
S	Off	60 min. Z1 (100+ rpm)	1:30 hr. Z1 to Z2
Totals: 11:30+ hr.	2:00+ hr.	5:00 hr.	4:30 hr.

WEEK 6	SWIM	BIKE	RUN
M	#16—Opt.	Rest day/slide day	Rest day/slide day
T	Off	Off	60 min. Z2 (at 10 min., insert 5 x 6 min. Z4 @ 3 min. jog)
W	#17	Trans: 45 min. Z2 (QC)	15 min. Z2
R	Off	60 min. Z2 (at 10 min., insert 8 x 3.5 min. Z4 Hill Repeats @ spin back down)	Off
F	#18	Off	60 min. Z2 (at 40 min., insert 15 min. Z4)
S	Off	Trans: 2:15 hr. Z2 (at 1:40, insert 30 min. Z4) (QC)	45 min. Z2
S	Off	60 min. Z1 (100+ rpm)	2:00 hr. Z1 to Z2
Totals: 12:00+ hr.	2:00+ hr.	5:00 hr.	5:00 hr.

WEEK 7	SWIM	BIKE	RUN
M	#19—Opt.	Rest day/slide day	Rest day/slide day
T	Off	Off	60 min. Z2 (at 10 min., insert 4 x 7.5 min. Z4 @ 3.5 min. jog)
W	#20	Trans: 45 min. Z2 (QC)	15 min. Z2
R	Off	60 min. Z2 (at 10 min., insert 2 x 7.5 min. Z4 @ 3.5 min. spin; then 3 x 5 min. Z4 @ 3 min. spin)	Off
F	#21	Off	60 min. Z2 (at 45 min., insert 10 min. Z4)
S	Off	Trans: 1:45 hr. Z2 (QC)	45 min. Z2
S	Off	30 min. Z1 (100+ rpm)	60 min. Z1 to Z2
Totals: 10:00+ hr.	2:00+ hr.	4:00 hr.	4:00 hr.

COMPETITIVE PROGRAM — SPRINT AND STANDARD DISTANCE TRIATHLONS

WEEK 8	SWIM	BIKE	RUN
M	Off	Rest day/slide day	Rest day/slide day
T	Off	Off	45 min. Z1 to Z2 (at 10 min., insert 5 x 1 min. PU @ 1 min. jog)
W	0.5 hr. easy	Trans: 45 min. Z1 to Z2 (QC)	15 min. Z1 to Z2
R	Off	60 min. Z1 (at 10 min., insert 5 x 1 min. PU @ 1 min. spin)	Off
F	0.5 hr. easy	Off	40 min. Z1 (at 10 min., insert 5 x 1 min. PU @ 1 min. jog)
S	Off	15 min. Z1—easy bike safety check	20 min. Z1—easy (in a.m.)
S	RACE!!!	RACE!!! (Sprint or Standard Distance Triathlon)	RACE!!! (Sprint or Standard Distance Triathlon)
Totals: 5:00+ hr.	1:00+ hr.	2:00 hr. (+Race)	2:00 hr. (+Race)

Swim Sessions for the Competitive Program

Our swims for the Competitive Program will all be approximately 3,000 yards or meters in length, which is a workout distance most athletes can complete within one hour. Our suggestion is that if you need to lengthen the session to last a full hour, simply extend the warm-up and/or cooldown portion as needed. If, however, you find you need to shorten the session to make it fit into an hour, reduce the main sets as needed but keep the warm-up, drills, and cooldown the same.

See page 112 for the numbered swim sessions to be used with this training program.

The second of our three eight-week training programs for the Sprint and Standard Distance Triathlon is the Intermediate Program.

Intermediate Training Program for Sprint and Standard Distance Triathlons

The Intermediate Program is for the athlete who fits best in between the Competitive Program and the Just-Finish Program, both in terms of time available to train and competitive goals. The Intermediate Program athlete needs to have available time to train for an average of about 7.5 hours a week, with several peak weeks of about ten hours. The total combined training time over the eight-week period is approximately sixty hours so we like to refer to this as the "sixty-hour plan."

If you are already in your racing season and in good form, you can begin the program immediately after your race. The first week is fully aerobic, which will help to complete your recovery and firm up your aerobic base. Then in the second week, we will include Easy Pickups on both the cycling and running sides to prepare us to transition into or higher-intensity sessions.

From there, our higher-intensity sessions and duration will build and become more challenging. We start at about 6.75 hours of training in the first week and then gradually build by about 45 minutes per week to about nine hours in the fourth week. This amount assumes two swims per week starting at about 45 minutes each in the first week and then increasing to one hour each in the fourth week.

Our quantity of Z4 training will gradually build and peak in week six at just over 75 minutes combined. Weeks three through six will each have three sessions that will include Z4 work, including two bike sessions and one run session. With five bike and/or run sessions per week during this period, this means that more than half of the sessions (60%) will include Z4 higher-intensity training.

Our longest sessions in the eight weeks will be three 2.5-hour transition sessions in weeks four, five, and six. Our longest runs of the eight weeks will be four 1.5-hour sessions in weeks three through six of the program.

With nine days to go before our race, we will transition into our crisp taper phase to have us rested, sharp, and race-ready. Our durations will gradually decrease and our intensities will be no higher than Z2 during these last nine days. At this point the hay is in the barn and it is time to taper smart and become physically and mentally energized.

If you are not coming off a race or you have not already built up to or close to 6.75 hours of training per week before starting the Intermediate

Program, it is suggested that you do. Depending on your starting point, complete four to eight weeks of moderate aerobic exercise to be properly prepared to begin the program. If you are starting from scratch, we suggest you start with two easy weekly swims of about 30 minutes each, three easy bike sessions of about 30 minutes each, and three easy run sessions of 15 to 30 minutes each. Then, over the four- to eight-week period, make gradual increases each week until you are comfortably up to or close to the 6.75-hour level. Once there, you are ready to begin with the first week of the eight-week program.

Intermediate Program

The following chart details the Eight-Week Intermediate Program.

INTERMEDIATE PROGRAM — SPRINT AND STANDARD DISTANCE TRIATHLONS

WEEK 1	SWIM	BIKE	RUN
M	#25— Opt.	Rest day/slide day	Rest day/slide day
T	Off	Off	45 min. Z2
W	#26	Trans: 45 min. Z2 (QC)	15 min. Z2
R	Off	45 min. Z2	Off
F	Or #25— Opt.	Off	Off
S	Off	Trans: 1:15 hr. Z2 (QC)	15 min. Z2
S	Off	Off	1:15 hr. Z1 to Z2
Totals: 6:45 hr.	1:30 hr.	2:45 hr.	2:30 hr.

WEEK 2	SWIM	BIKE	RUN
M	#27—Opt.	Rest day/slide day	Rest day/slide day
T	Off	Off	60 min. Z2 (at 10 min., insert 5 x 1 min. Easy Pickups @ 1 min. jog)
W	#28	Trans: 45 min. Z2 (QC)	15 min. Z2
R	Off	45 min. Z2 (at 10 min., insert 5 x 1 min. Easy Pickups @ 1 min. spin)	Off
F	Or #27—Opt.	Off	Off
S	Off	Trans: 1:30 hr. Z2 (at 1:15, insert 10 min. Z4) (QC)	30 min. Z2
S	Off	Off	1:15 hr. Z1 to Z2
Totals: 7:30 hr.	1:30 hr.	3:00 hr.	3:00 hr.

WEEK 3	SWIM	BIKE	RUN
M	#29—Opt.	Rest day/slide day	Rest day/slide day
T	Off	Off	60 min. Z2 (at 45 min., insert 5 min. Z4)
W	#30	Trans: 45 min. Z2 (QC)	15 min. Z2
R	Off	60 min. Z2 (at 10 min., insert 4 x 4 min. Z4 @ 2 min. spin; then 3 x 2 min. Z4 @ 1 min. spin)	Off
F	Or #29—Opt.	Off	Off
S	Off	Trans: 1:45 hr. Z2 (at 1:25, insert 15 min. Z4) (QC)	30 min. Z2
S	Off	Off	1:30 hr. Z1 to Z2
Totals: 8:15 hr.	1:30 hr.	3:30 hr.	3:15 hr.

WEEK 4	SWIM	BIKE	RUN
M	#45—Opt.	Rest day/slide day	Rest day/slide day
T	Off	Off	60 min. Z2 (at 10 min., insert 6 x 3 min. Z4 @ 1.5 min. jog)
W	#46	Trans: 45 min. Z2 (QC)	15 min. Z2
R	Off	60 min. Z2 (at 10 min., insert 10 x 2.5 min. Z4 Hill Repeats @ spin back down)	Off
F	Or #45—Opt.	Off	Off
S	Off	Trans: 2:00 hr. Z2 (at 1:35, insert 20 min. Z4) (QC)	30 min. Z2
S	Off	Off	1:30 hr. Z1 to Z2
Totals: 9:00 hr.	2:00 hr.	3:45 hr.	3:15 hr.

WEEK 5	SWIM	BIKE	RUN
M	#47—Opt.	Rest day/slide day	Rest day/slide day
T	Off	Off	60 min. Z2 (at 45 min., insert 10 min. Z4)
W	#48	Trans: 45 min. Z2 (QC)	15 min. Z2
R	Off	60 min. Z2 (at 10 min., insert 2 x 5 min. Z4 @ 3 min. spin; then 3 x 4 min. Z4 @ 2 min. spin)	Off
F	Or #47—Opt.	Off	Off
S	Off	Trans: 2:00 hr. Z2 (at 1:30, insert 25 min. Z4) (QC)	30 min. Z2
S	Off	Off	1:30 hr. Z1 to Z2
Totals: 9:00 hr.	2:00 hr.	3:45 hr.	3:15 hr.

WEEK 6	SWIM	BIKE	RUN
M	#49— Opt.	Rest day/slide day	Rest day/slide day
T	Off	Off	60 min. Z2 (at 10 min., insert 4 x 6 min. Z4 @ 3 min. jog)
W	#50	Trans: 45 min. Z2 (QC)	15 min. Z2
R	Off	60 min. Z2 (at 10 min., insert 8 x 3 min. Z4 Hill Repeats @ spin back down)	Off
F	Or #49— Opt.	Off	Off
S	Off	Trans: 2:00 hr. Z2 (at 1:25, insert 30 min. Z4) (QC)	30 min. Z2
S	Off	Off	1:30 hr. Z1 to Z2
Totals: 9:00 hr.	2:00 hr.	3:45 hr.	3:15 hr.

WEEK 7	SWIM	BIKE	RUN
M	#51— Opt.	Rest day/slide day	Rest day/slide day
T	Off	Off	60 min. Z2 (at 40 min., insert 15 min. Z4)
W	#52	Trans: 45 min. Z2 (QC)	15 min. Z2
R	Off	60 min. Z2 (at 10 min., insert 2 x 7.5 min. Z4 @ 3.5 min. spin; then 2 x 5 min. Z4 @ 3 min. spin)	Off
F	Or #51— Opt.	Off	Off
S	Off	Trans: 1:30 hr. Z2 (QC)	30 min. Z2
S	Off	Off	60 min. Z1 to Z2
Totals: 8:00 hr.	2:00 hr.	3:15 hr.	2:45 hr.

INTERMEDIATE PROGRAM — SPRINT AND STANDARD DISTANCE TRIATHLONS

WEEK 8	SWIM	BIKE	RUN
M	Off	Rest day/slide day	Rest day/slide day
T	Off	Off	45 min. Z1 to Z2 (at 10 min., insert 5 x 1 min. Easy Pickups @ 1 min. jog)
W	0.5 hr. easy	Trans: 45 min. Z1 to Z2 (QC)	15 min. Z1 to Z2
R	Off	60 min. Z1 (at 10 min., insert 5 x 1 min. Easy Pickups @ 1 min. spin)	Off
F	0.5 hr. easy	Off	Off
S	Off	15 min. Z1—easy bike safety check	30 min. Z1—easy (in a.m.)
S	RACE!!	RACE!!! (Sprint or Standard Distance Triathlon)	RACE!!! (Sprint or Standard Distance Triathlon)
Totals: 4:30+ hr.	1:00+ hr.	2:00 hr. (+Race)	1:30 hr. (+Race)

Swim Sessions for the Intermediate Program

Our swims through the first three weeks will all be approximately 2,000 yards or meters in length, which is a workout distance most athletes can complete within 45 minutes. Our swims will then increase to 2,500 yards or meters starting in the fourth week, which is a workout distance most athletes can complete in 60 minutes. Our suggestion is that if you need to lengthen the session to last a full 45 or 60 minutes, simply extend the warm-up and/or cooldown portion as needed. If, however, you find you need to shorten the session to make it fit into 45 or 60 minutes, reduce the main sets as needed, but keep the warm-up, drills, and cooldown the same.

See pages 114–115 for the numbered swim sessions to be used with this training program.

The final of our three eight-week training programs for the Sprint and Standard Distance Triathlon is the Just-Finish Program:

"Just-Finish" Training Program for Sprint and Standard Distance Triathlons

The Just-Finish Program is for the athlete who has limited time available to train, but would like to be able to complete a Sprint or Standard Distance Triathlon safely, in good health, and in good spirits. The Just-Finish athlete needs to have available time to train for an average of about five hours a week, with several peak weeks of about six hours. The total combined training time over the eight-week period is approximately forty hours so we like to refer to this as the "forty-hour plan."

If you are already in your racing season and in good form, you can begin the program immediately after your race. The first week is fully aerobic, which will help to complete your recovery and firm up your aerobic base. Then in the second week, we will include Easy Pickups on both the cycling and running sides to prepare us to transition into our higher-intensity sessions.

From there, our higher-intensity sessions and duration will build and become more challenging. We start at about four and a half hours of training in the first week and then gradually build by about 30 minutes per week to about six hours in the fourth week. This amount assumes two swims per week of about 45 minutes per session.

Our quantity of Z4 training will gradually build and peak in week six at just over 45 minutes combined. Weeks three through six will each have three sessions that will include Z4 work, including two bike sessions and one run session. With four bike and/or run sessions per week during this period, this means that more than half of the sessions (75 percent) will include Z4 higher-intensity training.

Our longest sessions in the eight weeks will be three two-hour transition sessions in weeks four, five, and six. Our longest runs of the eight weeks will be five one-hour sessions in weeks two through six of the program.

With nine days to go before our race, we will transition into our crisp taper-phase to have us rested, sharp, and race-ready. Our durations will gradually decrease and our intensities will be no higher than Z2 during these last nine days. At this point the hay is in the barn and it is time to taper smart and become physically and mentally energized.

If you are not coming off a race or you have not already built up to or close to 4.5 hours of training per week before starting the Just-Finish Program, it is suggested that you do. Depending on your starting point, complete four to eight weeks of moderate aerobic exercise to be properly prepared to begin the program. If you are starting from scratch, we suggest you start with two weekly easy swims of about 15 to 30 minutes each, two easy bike sessions of about 15 to 30 minutes each, and two easy run sessions of 15 to 30 minutes each. Then, over the four- to eight-week period, make gradual increases each week until you are comfortably up to or close to the 4.5-hour level. Once there, you are ready to begin with the first week of the eight-week program.

Just-Finish Program

The following chart details the Eight-Week Just-Finish Program.

JUST-FINISH PROGRAM — SPRINT AND STANDARD DISTANCE TRIATHLONS

WEEK 1	SWIM	BIKE	RUN
M	#25— Opt.	Rest day/slide day	Rest day/slide day
T	Off	45 min. Z2	Off
W	#26	Off	Off
R	Off	Off	45 min. Z2
F	Or #25— Opt.	Rest day/slide day	Rest day/slide day
S	Off	45 min. Z2	Off
S	Off	Off	45 min. Z1 to Z2
Totals: 4:30 hr.	1:30 hr.	1:30 hr.	1:30 hr.

WEEK 2	SWIM	BIKE	RUN
M	#27—Opt.	Rest day/slide day	Rest day/slide day
T	Off	45 min. Z2 (at 10 min., insert 5 x 1 min. Easy Pickups @ 1 min. spin)	Off
W	#28	Off	Off
R	Off	Off	45 min. Z2 (at 10 min., insert 5 x 1 min. Easy Pickups @ 1 min. jog)
F	Or #27—Opt.	Rest day/slide day	Rest day/slide day
S	Off	60 min. Z2 (at 45 min., insert 5 min. Z4)	Off
S	Off	Off	60 min. Z1 to Z2
Totals: 5:00 hr.	1:30 hr.	1:45 hr.	1:45 hr.

WEEK 3	SWIM	BIKE	RUN
M	#29—Opt.	Rest day/slide day	Rest day/slide day
T	Off	45 min. Z2 (at 10 min., insert 4 x 3 min. Z4 @ 1.5 min. spin)	Off
W	#30	Off	Off
R	Off	Off	45 min. Z2 (at 30 min., insert 5 min. Z4)
F	Or #29—Opt.	Rest day/slide day	Rest day/slide day
S	Off	Brick: 1:15 hr. Z2 (at 60 min., insert 10 min. Z4) (QC)	15 min. Z2
S	Off	Off	60 min. Z1 to Z2
Totals: 5:30 hr.	1:30 hr.	2:00 hr.	2:00 hr.

JUST-FINISH PROGRAM — SPRINT AND STANDARD DISTANCE TRIATHLON

WEEK 4	SWIM	BIKE	RUN
M	#31—Opt.	Rest day/slide day	Rest day/slide day
T	Off	45 min. Z2 (at 10 min., insert 7 x 2 min. Z4 Hill Repeats @ spin back down)	Off
W	#32	Off	Off
R	Off	Off	45 min. Z2 (at 30 min., insert 7.5 min. Z4)
F	Or #31—Opt.	Rest day/slide day	Rest day/slide day
S	Off	Brick: 1:30 hr. Z2 (at 1:10 hr., insert 15 min. Z4) (QC)	30 min. Z2
S	Off	Off	60 min. Z1 to Z2
Totals: 6:00 hr.	1:30 hr.	2:15 hr.	2:15 hr.

WEEK 5	SWIM	BIKE	RUN
M	#33—Opt.	Rest day/slide day	Rest day/slide day
T	Off	45 min. Z2 (at 10 min., insert 4 x 4 min. Z4 @ 2 min. spin)	Off
W	#34	Off	Off
R	Off	Off	45 min. Z2 (at 30 min., insert 10 min. Z4)
F	Or #33—Opt.	Rest day/slide day	Rest day/slide day
S	Off	Brick: 1:30 hr. Z2 (at 1:05 hr., insert 20 min. Z4) (QC)	30 min. Z2
S	Off	Off	60 min. Z1 to Z2
Totals: 6:00 hr.	1:30 hr.	2:15 hr.	2:15 hr.

WEEK 6	SWIM	BIKE	RUN
M	#35—Opt.	Rest day/slide day	Rest day/slide day
T	Off	45 min. Z2 (at 10 min., insert 6 x 2.5 min. Z4 Hill Repeats @ spin back down)	Off
W	#36	Off	Off
R	Off	Off	45 min. Z2 (at 25 min., insert 12.5 min. Z4)
F	Or #35—Opt.	Rest day/slide day	Rest day/slide day
S	Off	Brick: 1:30 hr. Z2 (at 1:05 hr., insert 20 min. Z4) (QC)	30 min. Z2
S	Off	Off	60 min. Z1 to Z2
Totals: 6:00 hr.	1:30 hr.	2:15 hr.	2:15 hr.

WEEK 7	SWIM	BIKE	RUN
M	#37—Opt.	Rest day/slide day	Rest day/slide day
T	Off	45 min. Z2 (at 10 min., insert 3 x 5 min. Z4 @ 3 min. spin)	Off
W	#38	Off	Off
R	Off	Off	45 min. Z2 (at 25 min., insert 15 min. Z4)
F	Or #37—Opt.	Rest day/slide day	Rest day/slide day
S	Off	Brick: 60 min. Z2 (QC)	15 min. Z2
S	Off	Off	45 min. Z1 to Z2
Totals: 5:00 hr.	1:30 hr.	1:45 hr.	1:45 hr.

JUST-FINISH PROGRAM — SPRINT AND STANDARD DISTANCE TRIATHLON

WEEK 8	SWIM	BIKE	RUN
M	Off	Rest day/slide day	Rest day/slide day
T	Off	45 min. Z2 (at 10 min., insert 5 x 1 min. Easy Pickups @ 1 min. spin)	Off
W	0.5 hr. easy	Off	Off
R	Off	Off	45 min. Z2 (at 10 min., insert 5 x 1 min. Easy Pickups @ 1 min. jog)
F	0.5 hr. easy	Rest day/slide day	Rest day/slide day
S	Off	30 min. Z1—easy bike safety check	30 min. Z1—easy (in a.m.)
S	RACE!!!	RACE!!! (Sprint/ Standard Distance Triathlon)	RACE!!! (Sprint/ Standard Distance Triathlon)
Totals: 3:30+ hr.	1:00+ hr.	1:15 hr. (+Race)	1:15 hr. (+Race)

Swim Sessions for the Just-Finish Program

Our swims sessions will all be approximately 2,000 yards or meters in length, which is a workout distance most athletes can complete within 45 minutes. Our suggestion is that if you need to lengthen the session to last 45 minutes, simply extend the warm-up and/or cooldown portion as needed. If, however, you find you need to shorten the session to make it fit into 45 minutes, reduce the main sets as needed, but keep the warm-up, drills, and cooldown the same.

See pages 114–115 for the numbered swim sessions to be used with this training program.

Guidelines for Adjusting the Sprint and Standard Distance Training Programs for Practice Races

It is not necessary to include any practice races prior to your Sprint or Standard Distance Triathlon. The benefits of appropriate practice races include preparing you to be race sharp, as well as helping to reduce nervousness and anxiety for your actual targeted race.

But if you do think you would like to include practice races, please consider the following suggestions.

Open-Water Swim: If you are a nervous swimmer or you haven't raced in open water in a while, an open-water swim race may be helpful. Swimming in open water and swimming in a crowd both take some getting used to. Also, if your race is going to have a wet suit–legal swim, this is an excellent opportunity to become used to swimming in a wet suit, if you are not already. Preferably, you will wear the same wet suit for your open-water swim as you plan to wear in your race.

We don't suggest tapering for this particular training race—instead just use it as a training session. Any distance up to 1 mile will do and it can be substituted for any of the planned swims. Since open-water swims are typically on Saturday or Sunday mornings, our suggestion is to simply complete it in the morning before your other bike and/or run training planned for that day and to count it toward any of your planned swim sessions. Any weekend between weeks two and seven is fine for this practice race, as long as you are at a point where you feel safe and comfortable in the open water.

Road Races: While not at all necessary, some athletes feel they benefit both physically and mentally from doing a road race prior to a Sprint or Standard Distance Triathlon. If you think you would like to do this, we suggest a 5K if you will be racing a Sprint triathlon and a 10K if you will be racing a Standard Distance Triathlon. The best time to include one of these races would be in the third through sixth weeks and to simply substitute them in as all or a portion of your weekly long-run session. We don't suggest tapering for this particular training race—instead just use it as a training session.

The **"Sprint to Standard" Approach:** Many athletes who have never raced a Standard Distance Triathlon will actually use a Sprint Distance Race as a tune-up race for the Standard Distance Triathlon. This approach works great, and if you decide to use it, we suggest you simply treat them as two separate races, using the eight-week program for the sprint and then going right back into the program after the sprint to prepare for the standard.

Adjusting Training Program for Missed Workouts

What if you miss a period of training due to an illness, a business trip, or some other reason? After not training for several days, we do not want to risk injury by immediately jumping back into our program where we left off. We want to ease back in safely at just the right rate of increase to get us back on track to achieving our goals.

Following are some guidelines on how to adjust your training for missed workouts.

Guidelines for Adjusting for Missed Workouts:

1. **One to two days missed training:** If you miss one to two days of training for any reason, and you cannot fit the missed sessions in by using the rest day/slide days, then just skip them. Missing one or two workouts is never going to matter in the long run, but trying to play catch-up by doubling up workouts is risky and could result in setbacks.

2. **Three to four days missed training:** Rejoin your training program (again, skip the missed days), but when you rejoin your program, do only half of the scheduled training on the first day back, and then resume full training on the second day back.

3. **Five to six days missed training:** Rejoin your training program (again, skip the missed days), but when you rejoin your program, do one-third of the scheduled training on the first two days back and two-thirds of the scheduled training on the next two days back. Resume full training of the fifth day back.

4. **Seven or more days missed training:** Reconsider the timing of your goal and consider a major redesign of your training program.

You should always first attempt to use the rest day/slide days to prevent missed workouts as discussed earlier. But if that is not possible to account for the missed workouts, please consider the above guidelines.

Other Training Program Adjustment Tips

Please consider the following additional training schedule adjustment tips.

The "mom shift": Don't forget to consider the "mom shift," which we discussed in Chapter 2. The training programs in this book are designed to best fit athletes who need to do their longest training sessions on Saturday and Sunday. If you find that other days work better for you—for example Tuesday and Wednesday—then consider shifting the entire weekly training cycle ahead by three days, so that the longer sessions fall on Tuesday and Wednesday.

Cross training through injury: If you miss training due to a minor injury, check with your doctor to see if a cross-training alternative can be substituted to keep you on schedule. For example, if your doctor determines that running will aggravate your injury, but the elliptical machine will not, consider substituting in elliptical sessions for your runs until you return to 100 percent good health.

Can I shorten the programs if I really only want to do sprints and not standards? While we really hope you will try to do the entire program even if you only plan to do sprints, the honest answer to this question is that you can get away with doing a little less to prepare for sprints if you really want to. Preparing for these two distances is so similar that the training is virtually the same. But you can still be ready for a sprint with a little less training time, especially if you are following the Just-Finish Program. If you are looking for places to cut training time off these programs because you really only want to "Just-Finish" a sprint, our suggestion is to decrease the length of one or both of the two longer weekend sessions.

Now that we have presented the three Sprint and Standard Distance Training programs, we will move on to Chapter 11, where we will present the Half Iron-Distance Training Program.

Training Programs for Half Iron-Distance Triathlons

This chapter includes three detailed Sixteen-Week Half Iron-Distance (approximately a 1.2-mile swim, 56-mile bike, and 13.1-mile run) training programs. Each program is based on the number of hours an athlete has available to train and level of competitiveness.

The Competitive Program includes approximately two hundred total training hours, with an average of about 12.5 hours per week and a maximum week of about 15.3 hours. The Intermediate Program has about 150 total training hours, with an average of about 9.4 hours per week and a maximum week of about 11.8 hours. The Just-Finish Program tops out at about one hundred total training hours, with an average of about 6.3 hours per week and a maximum week of about eight hours. The athlete simply selects the program that best fits her goals, competitiveness, level of experience, and available training time.

Each program tells the athlete exactly what to do each and every day throughout the eight-week period. There are none of the complicated formulas or overly general workout descriptions often found in other training books. Having worked with hundreds of female athletes for many years, we know that this is not what they want. Athletes want clear direction on exactly what they need to do and when. This is exactly what this chapter provides. The programs are designed to be efficient, productive, and enjoyable.

Following is a summary comparison of the three sixteen-week programs.

TRAINING PROGRAM	AVERAGE HOURS/WEEK	PEAK HOURS/WEEK	TOTAL HOURS (APPROX.)
Competitive	12.5	15.3	200
Intermediate	9.4	11.8	150
Just-Finish	6.3	8.0	100

You should consider the time management techniques presented in Chapter 2 and in the athlete profiles, and conservatively estimate your weekly training time availability. Once you have completed this analysis, simply select the program that best fits you, your goals, your experience level, and your available training time.

Each program starts with an eight-week base-building phase and then transitions into a second eight-week phase featuring higher-intensity training. Finally, each training program concludes with a nine-day pre-race taper phase to have you rested, sharp, and race-ready at just the right time for your Half Iron-Distance challenge.

Abbreviations for Training Programs

See page 110.

Notes to Swim Sessions in Training Programs

See page 111.

Following are our three Sixteen-Week Training Programs and full explanations of each, starting with the Sixteen-Week Competitive Program.

Competitive Sixteen-Week Training Program

The Competitive Program is for the experienced athlete who wants to maximize her potential and has available time to train for an average of about 12.5 hours a week, with several peak weeks of about 15.3 hours. The total combined training time over the sixteen-week period is approximately two hundred hours so we like to refer to this as the "200-hour plan."

The first eight weeks of the program contain the base-building phase. We start at about eight hours of fully aerobic (Z1 to Z2 heart rates) training in the first week and then gradually build by about one hour per week to about fifteen hours in the eighth week. This amount assumes two swims of about one hour per week, but this program also includes an optional third swim, which adds another hour to these totals. If swimming is your weakest of the three sports, it will be very helpful to include the third swim if possible.

If you have not already built up to or close to eight hours of training per week before starting the Competitive Program, it is suggested that you do.

Depending on your starting point, complete four to eight weeks of moderate aerobic exercise to be properly prepared to begin the program.

Our longest sessions in the first eight weeks will be a five-hour transition session and a 2.25-hour long run on the last weekend of the eighth week.

Base-Building Phase: Weeks One through Eight

The following chart details the eight-week base-building phase of the Competitive Program.

COMPETITIVE PROGRAM — BASE-BUILDING PHASE

WEEK 1	SWIM	BIKE	RUN
M	#1—Opt.	Rest day/slide day	Rest day/slide day
T	Off	Off	45 min. Z2
W	#2	Trans: 45 min. Z2 (QC)	15 min. Z2
R	Off	60 min. Z2	Off
F	#3	Off	45 min. Z2
S	Off	1:15 hr. Z2	Off
S	Off	30 min. Z1 (100+ rpm)	45 min. Z1 to Z2
Totals: 8:00+ hr.	2:00+ hr.	3:30 hr.	2:30 hr.

WEEK 2	SWIM	BIKE	RUN
M	#4—Opt.	Rest day/slide day	Rest day/slide day
T	Off	Off	45 min. Z2
W	#5	Trans: 45 min. Z2 (QC)	15 min. Z2
R	Off	60 min. Z2	Off
F	#6	Off	45 min. Z2
S	Off	Trans: 1:15 hr. Z2 (QC)	15 min. Z2
S	Off	60 min. Z1 (100+ rpm)	60 min. Z1 to Z2
Totals: 9:00+ hr.	2:00+ hr.	4:00 hr.	3:00 hr.

WEEK 3	SWIM	BIKE	RUN
M	#7—Opt.	Rest day/slide day	Rest day/slide day
T	Off	Off	45 min. Z2
W	#8	Trans: 45 min. Z2 (QC)	15 min. Z2
R	Off	60 min. Z2	Off
F	#9	Off	60 min. Z2
S	Off	Trans: 1:45 hr. Z2 (QC)	15 min. Z2
S	Off	60 min. Z1 (100+ rpm)	1:15 hr. Z1 to Z2
Totals: 10:00+ hr.	2:00+ hr.	4:30 hr.	3:30 hr.

COMPETITIVE PROGRAM — BASE-BUILDING PHASE

WEEK 4	SWIM	BIKE	RUN
M	#10—Opt.	Rest day/slide day	Rest day/slide day
T	Off	Off	45 min. Z2
W	#11	Trans: 45 min. Z2 (QC)	15 min. Z2
R	Off	60 min. Z2	Off
F	#12	Off	60 min. Z2
S	Off	Trans: 2:15 hr. Z2 (QC)	30 min. Z2
S	Off	60 min. Z1 (100+ rpm)	1:30 hr. Z1 to Z2
Totals: 11:00+ hr.	2:00+ hr.	5:00 hr.	4:00 hr.

WEEK 5	SWIM	BIKE	RUN
M	#13—Opt.	Rest day/slide day	Rest day/slide day
T	Off	Off	60 min. Z2
W	#14	Trans: 45 min. Z2 (QC)	15 min. Z2
R	Off	60 min. Z2	Off
F	#15	Off	60 min. Z2
S	Off	Trans: 2:45 hr. Z2 (QC)	30 min. Z2
S	Off	60 min. Z1 (100+ rpm)	1:45 hr. Z1 to Z2
Totals: 12:00+ hr.	2:00+ hr.	5:30 hr.	4:30 hr.

WEEK 6	SWIM	BIKE	RUN
M	#16—Opt.	Rest day/slide day	Rest day/slide day
T	Off	Off	60 min. Z2
W	#17	Trans: 45 min. Z2 (QC)	30 min. Z2
R	Off	60 min. Z2	Off
F	#18	Off	60 min. Z2
S	Off	Trans: 3:15 hr. Z2 (QC)	30 min. Z2
S	Off	60 min. Z1 (100+ rpm)	2:00 hr. Z1 to Z2
Totals: 13:00+ hr.	2:00+ hr.	6:00 hr.	5:00 hr.

WEEK 7	SWIM	BIKE	RUN
M	#19—Opt.	Rest day/slide day	Rest day/slide day
T	Off	Off	1:15 hr. Z2
W	#20	Trans: 45 min. Z2 (QC)	30 min. Z2
R	Off	60 min. Z2	Off
F	#21	Off	1:15 hr. Z2
S	Off	Trans: 3:45 hr. Z2 (QC)	45 min. Z2
S	Off	60 min. Z1 (100+ rpm)	1:45 hr. Z1 to Z2
Totals: 14:00+ hr.	2:00+ hr.	6:30 hr.	5:30 hr.

COMPETITIVE PROGRAM — BASE-BUILDING PHASE

WEEK 8	SWIM	BIKE	RUN
M	#22— Opt.	Rest day/slide day	Rest day/slide day
T	Off	Off	1:15 hr. Z2
W	#23	Trans: 45 min. Z2 (QC)	30 min. Z2
R	Off	60 min. Z2	Off
F	#24	Off	1:15 hr. Z2
S	Off	Trans: 4:15 hr. Z2 (QC)	45 min. Z2
S	Off	60 min. Z1 (100+ rpm)	2:15 hr. Z1 to Z2
Totals: 15:00+ hr.	2:00+ hr.	7:00 hr.	6:00 hr.

Swim Sessions for the Competitive Program

Our swims for the Competitive Program will be approximately 3,000 yards or meters in length, which is a workout distance most athletes can complete within one hour. Our suggestion is that if you need to lengthen the session to last a full hour, simply extend the warm-up and/or cooldown portions as needed. If, however, you find you need to shorten the session to make it fit into an hour, reduce the main sets as needed but keep the warm-up, drills, and cooldown the same.

See page 112 for the numbered swim sessions to be used with this training program.

Peak Training and Taper Phases: Weeks Nine through Sixteen

The second eight weeks (weeks nine through sixteen) of the Competitive Program include both the peak training phase and the taper phase. We start by including Easy Pickups in the ninth week to prepare us to introduce higher-intensity Z4 training. Our quantity of Z4 training will gradually build from there and peak in week fourteen. Weeks ten through fourteen will each have four sessions that will include Z4 work, including two bike sessions and two run sessions. With seven bike and/or run sessions per week during this period, this means that more than half of the sessions (57 percent) will include Z4 higher-intensity training.

During this second eight weeks, we will continue to include two swims of about one hour (3,000 yards/meters) each per week, with an optional third swim, which adds another hour to these totals. Again, if swimming is your weakest of the three triathlon sports, it will be very helpful to include the third swim if possible.

Just like in the first eight-week base-building phase, our longest sessions in the second eight weeks will be five-hour transition sessions and 2.25-hour long runs. This time, however, two of the five-hour transition sessions will be structured as "415-20-45 bricks" with 20-minute Z4 Inserts, and one will be structured with a 40-minute Z3 Insert (see Chapter 6).

With nine days to go before our Half Iron-Distance race, we will transition into our crisp taper phase to have us rested, sharp, and race-ready. Our durations will gradually decrease and our intensities will be no higher than Z2 during these last nine days. At this point the hay is in the barn and it is time to taper smart and become physically and mentally energized.

Following is the eight-week peak training and taper phase of the Competitive Program.

COMPETITIVE PROGRAM — PEAK TRAINING AND TAPER PHASES

WEEK 9	SWIM	BIKE	RUN
M	#2—Opt.	Rest day/slide day	Rest day/slide day
T	Off	Off	1:15 hr. Z2 (at 10 min. insert 5 x 1 min. PU @ 1 min. jog)
W	#1	Trans: 45 min. Z2 (QC)	30 min. Z2
R	Off	1:15 hr. Z2 (at 10 min., insert 5 x 1 min. PU @ 1 min. spin)	Off
F	#3	Off	1:15 hr. Z2 (at 60 min. insert 5 min. Z4)
S	Off	Trans: 4:15 hr. Z2 (at 4:00 hr. insert 5 min. Z4)(QC)	45 min. Z2
S	Off	60 min. Z1 (100+ rpm)	1:45 hr. Z1 to Z2
Totals: 14:45+ hr.	2:00+ hr.	7:15 hr.	5:30 hr.

WEEK 10	SWIM	BIKE	RUN
M	#5—Opt.	Rest day/slide day	Rest day/slide day
T	Off	Off	1:15 hr. Z2 (at 10 min. insert 10 x 2 min. Z4 @ 1 min. jog)
W	#4	Trans: 45 min. Z2 (QC)	30 min. Z2
R	Off	1:15 hr. Z2 (at 10 min., insert 10 x 2 min. Z4 Hill Repeats @ spin back down)	Off
F	#6	Off	1:15 hr. Z2 (at 60 min., insert 10 min. Z4)
S	Off	Trans: 4:15 hr. Z2 (at 4:00 hr. insert 10 min. Z4)(QC)	45 min. Z2
S	Off	60 min. Z1 (100+ rpm)	2:15 hr. Z1 to Z2
Totals: 15:15+ hr.	2:00+ hr.	7:15 hr.	6:00 hr.

WEEK 11	SWIM	BIKE	RUN
M	#8—Opt.	Rest day/slide day	Rest day/slide day
T	Off	Off	1:15 hr. Z2 (at 10 min. insert 8 x 3 min. Z4 @ 1.5 min. jog)
W	#7	Trans: 45 min. Z2 (QC)	30 min. Z2
R	Off	1:15 hr. Z2 (at 10 min., insert 7 x 4 min. Z4 @ 2 min. spin)	Off
F	#9	Off	1:15 hr. Z2 (at 55 min., insert 12.5 min. Z4)
S	Off	Trans: 4:15 hr. Z2 (at 3:55 hr., insert 15 min. Z4)(QC)	45 min. Z2
S	Off	60 min. Z1 (100+ rpm)	1:45 hr. Z1 to Z2
Totals: 14:45+ hr.	2:00+ hr.	7:15 hr.	5:30 hr.

WEEK 12	SWIM	BIKE	RUN
M	#11—Opt.	Rest day/slide day	Rest day/slide day
T	Off	Off	1:15 hr. Z2 (at 10 min. insert 6 x 4.5 min. Z4 @ 2 min. jog)
W	#10	Trans: 45 min. Z2 (QC)	30 min. Z2
R	Off	1:15 hr. Z2 (at 10 min., insert 12 x 2.5 min. Z4 Hill Repeats @ spin back down)	Off
F	#12	Off	1:15 hr. Z2 (at 55 min. insert 15 min. Z4)
S	Off	Trans: 4:15 hr. Z2 (at 3:50 hr. insert 20 min. Z4)(QC)	45 min. Z2
S	Off	60 min. Z1 (100+ rpm)	2:15 hr. Z1 to Z2
Totals: 15:15+ hr.	2:00+ hr.	7:15 hr.	6:00 hr.

COMPETITIVE PROGRAM — PEAK TRAINING AND TAPER PHASES

WEEK 13	SWIM	BIKE	RUN
M	#14—Opt.	Rest day/slide day	Rest day/slide day
T	Off	Off	1:15 hr. Z2 (at 10 min. insert 5 x 6 min. Z4 @ 3 min. jog)
W	#13	Trans: 45 min. Z2 (QC)	30 min. Z2
R	Off	1:15 hr. Z2 (at 10 min., insert 6 x 5 min. Z4 @ 2.5 min. spin)	Off
F	#15	Off	1:15 hr. Z2 (at 15 min. insert 15 min. Z4)
S	Off	Trans: 4:15 hr. Z2 (at 3:50 hrs insert 20 min. Z4)(QC)	45 min. Z2
S	Off	60 min. Z1 (100+ rpm)	1:45 hr. Z1 to Z2
Totals: 14:45+ hr.	2:00+ hr.	7:15 hr.	5:30 hr.

WEEK 14	SWIM	BIKE	RUN
M	#17—Opt.	Rest day/slide day	Rest day/slide day
T	Off	Off	1:15 hr. Z2 (at 10 min. insert 4 x 7.5 min. Z4 @ 3.5 min. jog)
W	#16	Trans: 45 min. Z2 (QC)	30 min. Z2
R	Off	1:15 hr. Z2 (at 10 min. insert 10 x 3 min. Z4 Hill Repeats @ spin back down)	Off
F	#18	Off	1:15 hr. Z2 (at 55 min., insert 15 min. Z4)
S	Off	Trans: 4:15 hr. Z2 (at 3:30 hr. insert 40 min. Z3) (QC)	45 min. Z2
S	Off	60 min. Z1 (100+ rpm)	2:15 hr. Z1 to Z2
Totals: 15:15+ hr.	2:00+ hr.	7:15 hr.	6:00 hr.

WEEK 15	SWIM	BIKE	RUN
M	#20—Opt.	Rest day/slide day	Rest day/slide day
T	Off	Off	1:15 hr. Z2 (at 10 min. insert 1 x 10 min. Z4 @ 5 min. jog, then 10 x 2 min. Z4 @ 1 min. jog)
W	#19	Trans: 45 min. Z2 (QC)	30 min. Z2
R	Off	1:15 hr. Z2 (at 10 min., insert 4 x 7.5 min. Z4 @ 3.5 min. spin)	Off
F	#21	Off	1:15 hr. Z2 (at 60 min. insert 10 min. Z4)
S	Off	Trans: 2:15 hr. Z2 (QC)	30 min. Z2
S	Off	45 min. Z1 (100+ rpm)	60 min. Z1 to Z2
Totals: 11:30+ hr.	2:00+ hr.	5:00 hr.	4:30 hr.

WEEK 16	SWIM	BIKE	RUN
M	Off	Rest day/slide day	Rest day/slide day
T	Off	Off	45 min. Z1 to Z2 (at 10 min. insert 5 x 1 min. PU @ 1 min. jog)
W	0.5 hr. easy	Trans: 45 min. Z1 to Z2 (QC)	15 min. Z1 to Z2
R	Off	60 min. Z1 (at 10 min. insert 5 x 1 min. PU @ 1 min. spin)	Off
F	0.5 hr. easy	Off	40 min. Z1 (at 10 min., insert 5 x 1 min. PU @ 1 min. jog)
S	Off	15 min. Z1—easy bike safety check	20 min. Z1—easy (in a.m.)
S	Race!! Half Iron-Distance	Race!! Half Iron-Distance	Race!! Half Iron-Distance
Totals: 5:00+ hr.	1:00 hr. (+R)	2:00 hr. (+Race)	2:00 hr. (+Race)

The second of our three sixteen-week training programs is the Intermediate Program.

Intermediate Sixteen-Week Training Program

The Intermediate Program is for the athlete who fits best in between the Competitive Program and the Just-Finish Program, both in terms of time available to train and competitive goals. The Intermediate Program athlete needs to have available time to train for an average of about 9.4 hours a week, with several peak weeks of about 11.8 hours. The total combined training time over the sixteen-week period is about 150 hours, so we like to refer to this one as the "150-hour plan."

The first eight weeks of the program is the base-building phase. We start at about six hours of fully aerobic (Z1 to Z2 heart rates) training in the first week and then gradually build by about 45 minutes per week to about eleven hours in the eighth week. This amount assumes two swims of about 45 minutes per week.

If you have not already built up to or close to six hours of training per week before starting the Intermediate Program, it is suggested that you do. Depending on your starting point, complete four to eight weeks of moderate aerobic exercise to be properly prepared to begin the program.

Our longest sessions in the first eight weeks will be a 4.5-hour transition session and a 2.25-hour long run on the last weekend of the eighth week.

Base-Building Phase: Weeks One through Eight
The following chart details the eight-week base-building phase of the Intermediate Program.

INTERMEDIATE PROGRAM — BASE-BUILDING PHASE

WEEK 1	SWIM	BIKE	RUN
M	Rest day/ slide day	Rest day/slide day	Rest day/slide day
T	#25	Off	45 min. Z2
W	Off	Trans: 30 min. Z2 (QC)	15 min. Z2
R	#26	45 min. Z2	Off
F	Rest day/ slide day	Rest day/slide day	Rest day/slide day
S	Off	1:15 hr. Z2	Off
S	Off	Off	60 min. Z1 to Z2
Totals: 6:00 hr.	1:30 hr.	2:30 hr.	2:00 hr.

WEEK 2	SWIM	BIKE	RUN
M	Rest day/ slide day	Rest day/slide day	Rest day/slide day
T	#27	Off	45 min. Z2
W	Off	Trans: 30 min. Z2 (QC)	15 min. Z2
R	#28	45 min. Z2	Off
F	Rest day/ slide day	Rest day/slide day	Rest day/slide day
S	Off	1:45 hr. Z2	Off
S	Off	Off	1:15 hr. Z1 to Z2
Totals: 6:45 hr.	1:30 hr.	3:00 hr.	2:15 hr.

INTERMEDIATE PROGRAM — BASE-BUILDING PHASE

WEEK 3	SWIM	BIKE	RUN
M	Rest day/ slide day	Rest day/slide day	Rest day/slide day
T	#29	Off	45 min. Z2
W	Off	Trans: 45 min. Z2 (QC)	15 min. Z2
R	#30	45 min. Z2	Off
F	Rest day/ slide day	Rest day/slide day	Rest day/slide day
S	Off	Trans: 1:45 hr. Z2 (QC)	15 min. Z2
S	Off	Off	1:30 hr. Z1 to Z2
Totals: 7:30 hr.	1:30 hr.	3:15 hr.	2:45 hr.

WEEK 4	SWIM	BIKE	RUN
M	Rest day/ slide day	Rest day/slide day	Rest day/slide day
T	#31	Off	45 min. Z2
W	Off	Trans: 45 min. Z2 (QC)	15 min. Z2
R	#32	60 min. Z2	Off
F	Rest day/ slide day	Rest day/slide day	Rest day/slide day
S	Off	Trans: 2:15 hr. Z2 (QC)	15 min. Z2
S	Off	Off	1:30 hr. Z1 to Z2
Totals: 8:15 hr.	1:30 hr.	4:00 hr.	2:45 hr.

WEEK 5	SWIM	BIKE	RUN
M	Rest day/ slide day	Rest day/slide day	Rest day/slide day
T	#33	Off	60 min. Z2
W	Off	Trans: 45 min. Z2 (QC)	15 min. Z2
R	#34	60 min. Z2	Off
F	Rest day/ slide day	Rest day/slide day	Rest day/slide day
S	Off	Trans: 2:45 hr. Z2 (QC)	15 min. Z2
S	Off	Off	1:30 hr. Z1 to Z2
Totals: 9:00 hr.	1:30 hr.	4:30 hr.	3:00 hr.

WEEK 6	SWIM	BIKE	RUN
M	Rest day/ slide day	Rest day/slide day	Rest day/slide day
T	#35	Off	60 min. Z2
W	Off	Trans: 45 min. Z2 (QC)	15 min. Z2
R	#36	60 min. Z2	Off
F	Rest day/ slide day	Rest day/slide day	Rest day/slide day
S	Off	Trans: 3:15 hr. Z2 (QC)	15 min. Z2
S	Off	Off	1:45 hr. Z1 to Z2
Totals: 9:45 hr.	1:30 hr.	5:00 hr.	3:15 hr.

INTERMEDIATE PROGRAM — BASE-BUILDING PHASE

WEEK 7	SWIM	BIKE	RUN
M	Rest day/ slide day	Rest day/slide day	Rest day/slide day
T	#37	Off	60 min. Z2
W	Off	Trans: 45 min. Z2 (QC)	15 min. Z2
R	#38	60 min. Z2	Off
F	Rest day/ slide day	Rest day/slide day	Rest day/slide day
S	Off	Trans: 3:45 hr. Z2 (QC)	15 min. Z2
S	Off	Off	2:00 hr. Z1 to Z2
Totals: 10:30 hr.	1:30 hr.	5:30 hr.	3:30 hr.
WEEK 8	**SWIM**	**BIKE**	**RUN**
M	Rest day/ slide day	Rest day/slide day	Rest day/slide day
T	#39	Off	60 min. Z2
W	Off	Trans: 45 min. Z2 (QC)	15 min. Z2
R	#40	60 min. Z2	Off
F	Rest day/ slide day	Rest day/slide day	Rest day/slide day
S	Off	Trans: 4:15 hr. Z2 (QC)	15 min. Z2
S	Off	Off	2:15 hr. Z1 to Z2
Totals: 11:15 hr.	1:30 hr.	6:00 hr.	3:45 hr.

Swim Sessions for the Intermediate Program

Our swims through the first eight weeks will all be approximately 2,000 yards or meters in length, which is a workout distance most athletes can complete within 45 minutes. Our suggestion is that if you need to lengthen the session to last a full 45 minutes, simply extend the warm-up and/or cooldown portions as needed. If, however, you find you need to shorten the session to make it fit into 45 minutes, reduce the main sets as needed, but keep the warm-up, drills, and cooldown the same.

See page 114 for the numbered swim sessions to be used with this training program.

Peak Training and Taper Phases: Weeks Nine through Sixteen

The second eight weeks (weeks nine through sixteen) of the Intermediate Program include both the peak training phase and the taper phase. We start by including Easy Pickups in the ninth week to prepare us to introduce higher-intensity Z4 training. Our quantity of Z4 training will gradually build from there and peak in week fourteen. Weeks ten through fourteen will each have three sessions that will include Z4 work, including two bike sessions and one run session. With five bike and/or run sessions per week during this period, this means that more than half of the sessions (60%) will include Z4 higher-intensity training.

During this phase we will continue to include two swims each week, but each session will now increase to about 2,500 yards/meters.

Our longest sessions in the second eight weeks will be five-hour transition sessions and 2.25-hour long runs. This time, however, one of the long transition sessions will be structured as a "415-20-45 brick" with a 20-minute Z4 Insert and one will be structured with a 40-minute Z3 Insert.

With nine days to go before our Half Iron-Distance race, we will transition into our crisp taper phase to have us rested, sharp, and race-ready. Our volumes will gradually decrease and our intensities will be no higher than Z2 during these last nine days. At this point the hay is in the barn and it is time to taper smart and become physically and mentally energized.

Following is the eight-week peak training phase and taper phase of the Intermediate Program.

INTERMEDIATE PROGRAM — PEAK TRAINING AND TAPER PHASES

WEEK 9	SWIM	BIKE	RUN
M	Rest day/ slide day	Rest day/slide day	Rest day/slide day
T	#45	Off	60 min. Z2 (at 10 min., insert 5 x 1 min. PU @ 1 min. jog)
W	Off	Trans: 45 min. Z2 (QC)	15 min. Z2
R	#46	60 min. Z2 (at 10 min., insert 5 x 1 min. PU @ 1 min. spin)	Off
F	Rest day/ slide day	Rest day/slide day	Rest day/slide day
S	Off	Trans: 4:15 hr. Z2 (at 4:00 hr. insert 5 min. Z4) (QC)	45 min. Z2
S	Off	Off	1:45 hr. Z1 to Z2
Totals: 11:45 hr.	2:00 hr.	6:00 hr.	3:45 hr.

WEEK 10	SWIM	BIKE	RUN
M	Rest day/ slide day	Rest day/slide day	Rest day/slide day
T	#47	Off	60 min. Z2 (at 10 min., insert 10 x 2 min. Z4 @ 1 min. jog)
W	Off	Trans: 45 min. Z2 (QC)	15 min. Z2
R	#48	60 min. Z2 (at 10 min., insert 10 x 2 min. Z4 Hill Repeats @ spin back down)	Off
F	Rest day/ slide day	Rest day/slide day	Rest day/slide day
S	Off	Trans: 3:15 hr. Z2 (at 3:00 hr. insert 10 min. Z4) (QC)	15 min. Z2
S	Off	30 min. Z1 (100+ rpm)	2:15 hr. Z1 to Z2
Totals: 11:15 hr.	2:00 hr.	5:30 hr.	3:45 hr.

WEEK 11	SWIM	BIKE	RUN
M	Rest day/slide day	Rest day/slide day	Rest day/slide day
T	#49	Off	60 min. Z2 (at 45 min., insert 10 min. Z4)
W	Off	Trans: 45 min. Z2 (QC)	15 min. Z2
R	#50	60 min. Z2 (at 10 min., insert 6 x 4 min. Z4 @ 2 min. spin)	Off
F	Rest day/slide day	Rest day/slide day	Rest day/slide day
S	Off	Trans: 4:15 hr. Z2 (at 3:55 hr. insert 15 min. Z4) (QC)	45 min. Z2
S	Off	Off	1:45 hr. Z1 to Z2
Totals: 11:45 hr.	2:00 hr.	6:00 hr.	3:45 hr.

WEEK 12	SWIM	BIKE	RUN
M	Rest day/slide day	Rest day/slide day	Rest day/slide day
T	#51	Off	60 min. Z2 (at 10 min., insert 8 x 3 min. Z4 @ 1.5 min. jog)
W	Off	Trans: 45 min. Z2 (QC)	15 min. Z2
R	#52	60 min. Z2 (at 10 min., insert 10 x 2.5 min. Z4 Hill Repeats @ spin back down)	Off
F	Rest day/slide day	Rest day/slide day	Rest day/slide day
S	Off	Trans: 3:15 hr. Z2 (at 2:50 hr. insert 20 min. Z4) (QC)	15 min. Z2
S	Off	30 min. Z1 (100+ rpm)	2:15 hr. Z1 to Z2
Totals: 11:15 hr.	2:00 hr.	5:30 hr.	3:45 hr.

INTERMEDIATE PROGRAM — PEAK TRAINING AND TAPER PHASES

WEEK 13	SWIM	BIKE	RUN
M	Rest day/ slide day	Rest day/slide day	Rest day/slide day
T	#53	Off	60 min. Z2 (at 40 min., insert 12.5 min. Z4)
W	Off	Trans: 45 min. Z2 (QC)	15 min. Z2
R	#54	60 min. Z2 (at 10 min., insert 5 x 5 min. Z4 @ 2.5 min. spin)	Off
F	Rest day/ slide day	Rest day/slide day	Rest day/slide day
S	Off	Trans: 4:15 hr. Z2 (at 3:50 hr. insert 20 min. Z4) (QC)	45 min. Z2
S	Off	Off	1:45 hr. Z1 to Z2
Totals: 11:45 hr.	2:00 hr.	6:00 hr.	3:45 hr.

WEEK 14	SWIM	BIKE	RUN
M	Rest day/ slide day	Rest day/slide day	Rest day/slide day
T	#55	Off	60 min. Z2 (at 10 min., insert 4 x 6 min. Z4 @ 3 min. jog)
W	Off	Trans: 45 min. Z2 (QC)	15 min. Z2
R	#56	60 min. Z2 (at 10 min., insert 8 x 3 min. Z4 Hill Repeats @ spin back down)	Off
F	Rest day/ slide day	Rest day/slide day	Rest day/slide day
S	Off	Trans: 3:15 hr. Z2 (at 2:30 hr. insert 40 min. Z3)(QC)	15 min. Z2
S	Off	30 min. Z1 (100+ rpm)	2:15 hr. Z1 to Z2
Totals: 11:15 hr.	2:00 hr.	5:30 hr.	3:45 hr.

WEEK 15	SWIM	BIKE	RUN
M	Rest day/ slide day	Rest day/slide day	Rest day/slide day
T	#57	Off	60 min. Z2 (at 40 min., insert 15 min. Z4)
W	Off	Trans: 45 min. Z2 (QC)	15 min. Z2
R	#58	60 min. Z2 (at 10 min., insert 3 x 7.5 min. Z4 @ 3.5 min. spin)	Off
F	Rest day/ slide day	Rest day/slide day	Rest day/slide day
S	Off	Trans: 2:15 hr. Z2 (QC)	15 min. Z2
S	Off	30 min. Z1 (100+ rpm)	60 min. Z1 to Z2
Totals: 9:00 hr.	2:00 hr.	4:30 hr.	2:30 hr.

WEEK 16	SWIM	BIKE	RUN
M	Rest day/ slide day	Rest day/slide day	Rest day/slide day
T	0.5 hr. easy	Off	45 min. Z1 to Z2 (at 10 min., insert 5 x 1 min. PU @ 1 min. jog)
W	Off	Trans: 45 min. Z1 to Z2 (QC)	15 min. Z1 to Z2
R	0.5 hr. easy	60 min. Z1 (at 10 min., insert 5 x 1 min. PU @ 1 min. spin)	Off
F	Off	Off	40 min. Z1 (at 10 min., insert 5 x 1 min. PU @ 1 min. jog)
S	Off	15 min. Z1—easy bike safety check	20 min. Z1—easy (in a.m.)
S	Race!! Half Iron-Distance	Race!! Half Iron-Distance	Race!! Half Iron-Distance
Totals: 5:00+ hr.	1:00 hr. (+R)	2:00 hr. (+Race)	2:00 hr. (+Race)

The final of our three sixteen-week training programs is the Just-Finish Program.

Just-Finish Sixteen-Week Training Program

The Just-Finish Program is for the athlete who has limited time available to train but would like to be able to complete the Half Iron-Distance Triathlon safely, in good health, and in good spirits. The Just-Finish Program athlete needs to have available time to train for an average of about 6.3 hours a week, with several peak weeks of about eight hours. The total combined training time over the sixteen-week period is approximately one hundred hours, so we like to refer to this as the "100-hour plan."

The first eight weeks of the program are the base-building phase. We start at about four hours of fully aerobic (Z1 to Z2 heart rates) training in the first week and then gradually build by about 30 minutes per week to about 7.5 hours in the eighth week. This amount assumes two swims of about 45 minutes each per week.

If you have not already built up to or close to four hours of training per week before starting the Just-Finish Program, it is suggested that you do. Depending on your starting point, complete four to eight weeks of moderate aerobic exercise to be properly prepared to begin the program.

Our longest sessions in the first eight weeks will be a two-hour bike session and a 1.75-hour long run on the last weekend of the eighth week.

Base-Building Phase: Weeks One through Eight

The following chart details the eight-week base-building phase of the Just-Finish Program.

JUST-FINISH PROGRAM — BASE-BUILDING PHASE

WEEK 1	SWIM	BIKE	RUN
M	Rest day/ slide day	Rest day/slide day	Rest day/slide day
T	#25	Off	30 min. Z2
W	Off	Trans: 15 min. Z2 (QC)	15 min. Z2
R	#26	30 min. Z2	Off
F	Rest day/ slide day	Rest day/slide day	Rest day/slide day
S	Off	30 min. Z2	Off
S	Off	Off	30 min. Z1 to Z2
Totals: 4:00 hr.	1:30 hr.	1:15 hr.	1:15 hr.
WEEK 2	SWIM	BIKE	RUN
M	Rest day/ slide day	Rest day/slide day	Rest day/slide day
T	#27	Off	30 min. Z2
W	Off	Trans: 30 min. Z2 (QC)	15 min. Z2
R	#28	30 min. Z2	Off
F	Rest day/ slide day	Rest day/slide day	Rest day/slide day
S	Off	30 min. Z2	Off
S	Off	Off	45 min. Z1 to Z2
Totals: 4:30 hr.	1:30 hr.	1:30 hr.	1:30 hr.

JUST-FINISH PROGRAM — BASE-BUILDING PHASE

WEEK 3	SWIM	BIKE	RUN
M	Rest day/ slide day	Rest day/slide day	Rest day/slide day
T	#29	Off	45 min. Z2
W	Off	Trans: 30 min. Z2 (QC)	15 min. Z2
R	#30	30 min. Z2	Off
F	Rest day/ slide day	Rest day/slide day	Rest day/slide day
S	Off	45 min. Z2	Off
S	Off	Off	45 min. Z1 to Z2
Totals: 5:00 hr.	1:30 hr.	1:45 hr.	1:45 hr.

WEEK 4	SWIM	BIKE	RUN
M	Rest day/ slide day	Rest day/slide day	Rest day/slide day
T	#31	Off	45 min. Z2
W	Off	Trans: 30 min. Z2 (QC)	15 min. Z2
R	#32	30 min. Z2	Off
F	Rest day/ slide day	Rest day/slide day	Rest day/slide day
S	Off	60 min. Z2	Off
S	Off	Off	1:00 hr. Z1 to Z2
Totals: 5:30 hr.	1:30 hr.	2:00 hr.	2:00 hr.

WEEK 5	SWIM	BIKE	RUN
M	Rest day/ slide day	Rest day/slide day	Rest day/slide day
T	#33	Off	45 min. Z2
W	Off	Trans: 30 min. Z2 (QC)	15 min. Z2
R	#34	45 min. Z2	Off
F	Rest day/ slide day	Rest day/slide day	Rest day/slide day
S	Off	1:15 hr. Z2	Off
S	Off	Off	60 min. Z1 to Z2
Totals: 6:00 hr.	1:30 hr.	2:30 hr.	2:00 hr.

WEEK 6	SWIM	BIKE	RUN
M	Rest day/ slide day	Rest day/slide day	Rest day/slide day
T	#35	Off	45 min. Z2
W	Off	Trans: 30 min. Z2 (QC)	15 min. Z2
R	#36	45 min. Z2	Off
F	Rest day/ slide day	Rest day/slide day	Rest day/slide day
S	Off	1:30 hr. Z2	Off
S	Off	Off	1:15 hr. Z1 to Z2
Totals: 6:30 hr.	1:30 hr.	2:45 hr.	2:15 hr.

JUST-FINISH PROGRAM — BASE-BUILDING PHASE

WEEK 7	SWIM	BIKE	RUN
M	Rest day/ slide day	Rest day/slide day	Rest day/slide day
T	#37	Off	45 min. Z2
W	Off	Trans: 30 min. Z2 (QC)	15 min. Z2
R	#38	45 min. Z2	Off
F	Rest day/ slide day	Rest day/slide day	Rest day/slide day
S	Off	2:00 hr. Z2	Off
S	Off	Off	1:15 hr. Z1 to Z2
Totals: 7:00 hr.	1:30 hr.	3:15 hr.	2:15 hr.
WEEK 8	**SWIM**	**BIKE**	**RUN**
M	Rest day/ slide day	Rest day/slide day	Rest day/slide day
T	#39	Off	45 min. Z2
W	Off	Trans: 30 min. Z2 (QC)	15 min. Z2
R	#40	45 min. Z2	Off
F	Rest day/ slide day	Rest day/slide day	Rest day/slide day
S	Off	2:00 hr. Z2	Off
S	Off	Off	1:45 hr. Z1 to Z2
Totals: 7:30 hr.	1:30 hr.	3:15 hr.	2:45 hr.

Swim Sessions for the Just-Finish Program

Our swims for the Just-Finish Program will all be approximately 2,000 yards or meters in length, which is a workout distance most athletes can complete within 45 minutes. Our suggestion is that if you need to lengthen the session to last 45 minutes, simply extend the warm-up and/or cooldown portions as needed. If, however, you find you need to shorten the session to make it fit into 45 minutes, reduce the main sets as needed, but keep the warm-up, drills, and cooldown the same.

See page 114 for the numbered swim sessions to be used with this training program.

Peak Training and Taper Phases: Weeks Nine through Sixteen

The second eight weeks (weeks nine through sixteen) of the Just-Finish Program include both the peak training and the taper phase. We start by including Easy Pickups in the ninth week to prepare us to introduce higher-intensity Z4 training. Our quantity of Z4 training will gradually build from there and peak in week fourteen. Weeks ten through fourteen will each have three sessions that will include Z4 work, including two bike sessions and one run session. With five bike and/or run sessions per week during this period, this means that more than half of the sessions (60 percent) will include Z4 higher-intensity training.

During this phase we will continue to include two swims of about 45 minutes (2,000 yards/meters) each per week.

Our longest sessions in the second eight weeks will be 3.5-hour transition sessions and 2.25-hour long runs. One of the 3.5-hour transition sessions will be structured as a shorter version of a "415-20-45 brick" with a 20-minute Z4 Insert.

With nine days to go before our Half Iron-Distance race, we will transition into our crisp taper phase to have us rested, sharp, and race-ready. Our volumes will gradually decrease and our intensities will be no higher than Z2 during these last nine days. At this point the hay is in the barn and it is time to taper smart and become physically and mentally energized.

Following is the eight-week peak training and taper phase of the Just-Finish Program.

JUST-FINISH PROGRAM — PEAK TRAINING AND TAPER PHASES

WEEK 9	SWIM	BIKE	RUN
M	Rest day/ slide day	Rest day/slide day	Rest day/slide day
T	#41	Off	45 min. Z2 (at 10 min., insert 5 x 1 min. PU @ 1 min. jog)
W	Off	Trans: 30 min. Z2 (QC)	15 min. Z2
R	#42	45 min. Z2 (at 10 min., insert 5 x 1 min. PU@ 1 min. spin)	Off
F	Rest day/ slide day	Rest day/slide day	Rest day/slide day
S	Off	Trans: 2:45 hr. Z2 (at 2:30 hrs. insert 5 min. Z4)(QC)	15 min. Z2
S	Off	Off	1:15 hr. Z1 to Z2
Totals: 8:00 hr.	1:30 hr.	4:00 hr.	2:30 hr.

WEEK 10	SWIM	BIKE	RUN
M	Rest day/ slide day	Rest day/slide day	Rest day/slide day
T	#43	Off	45 min. Z2 (at 10 min., 6 x 2 min. Z4 @1 min. jog)
W	Off	Trans: 30 min. Z2 (QC)	15 min. Z2
R	#44	45 min. Z2 (at 10 min., 6 x 2 min. Z4 Hill Repeats @ spin back down)	Off
F	Rest day/ slide day	Rest day/slide day	Rest day/slide day
S	Off	Trans: 60 min. Z2 (at 45 min., insert 10 min. Z4)(QC)	15 min. Z2
S	Off	Opt.: 30 min. Z1 (100+ rpm)	2:00 hr. Z1 to Z2
Totals: 7:00+ hr.	1:30 hr.	2:15+ hr.	3:15 hr.

WEEK 11	SWIM	BIKE	RUN
M	Rest day/ slide day	Rest day/slide day	Rest day/slide day
T	#25	Off	45 min. Z2 (at 30 min., insert 10 min. Z4)
W	Off	Trans: 30 min. Z2 (QC)	15 min. Z2
R	#26	45 min. Z2 (at 10 min., insert 5 x 4 min. Z4 @ 2 min. spin)	Off
F	Rest day/ slide day	Rest day/slide day	Rest day/slide day
S	Off	Trans: 3:15 hr. Z2 (at 2:55 hr. insert 15 min. Z4) (QC)	15 min. Z2
S	Off	Off	45 min. Z1 to Z2
Totals: 8:00 hr.	1:30 hr.	4:30 hr.	2:00 hr.
WEEK 12	SWIM	BIKE	RUN
M	Rest day/ slide day	Rest day/slide day	Rest day/slide day
T	#27	Off	45 min. Z2 (at 10 min., insert 5 x 3 min. Z4 @ 1.5 min. jog)
W	Off	Trans: 30 min. Z2 (QC)	15 min. Z2
R	#28	45 min. Z2 (at 10 min., insert 6 x 2.5 min. Z4 Hill Repeats @ spin back down)	Off
F	Rest day/ slide day	Rest day/slide day	Rest day/slide day
S	Off	Trans: 45 min. Z2 (at 20 min. insert 20 min. Z4) (QC)	15 min. Z2
S	Off	Opt: 30 min. Z1 (100+ rpm)	2:15 hr. Z1 to Z2
Totals: 7:00+ hr.	1:30 hr.	2:00+ hr.	3:30 hr.

WEEK 13	SWIM	BIKE	RUN
M	Rest day/ slide day	Rest day/slide day	Rest day/slide day
T	#29	Off	45 min. Z2 (at 25 min., insert 12.5 min. Z4)
W	Off	Trans: 30 min. Z2 (QC)	15 min. Z2
R	#30	45 min. Z2 (at 10 min., insert 4 x 5 min. Z4 @ 3 min. spin)	Off
F	Rest day/ slide day	Rest day/slide day	Rest day/slide day
S	Off	Trans: 3:15 hr. Z2 (at 2:50 hr., insert 20 min. Z4)(QC)	15 min. Z2
S	Off	Off	45 min. Z1 to Z2
Totals: 8:00 hr.	1:30 hr.	4:30 hr.	2:00 hr.

WEEK 14	SWIM	BIKE	RUN
M	Rest day/ slide day	Rest day/slide day	Rest day/slide day
T	#31	Off	45 min. Z2 (at 10 min., insert 3 x 6 min. Z4 @ 3 min. jog)
W	Off	Trans: 30 min. Z2 (QC)	15 min. Z2
R	#32	45 min. Z2 (at 10 min., insert 6 x 3 min. Z4 Hill Repeats @ spin back down)	Off
F	Rest day/ slide day	Rest day/slide day	Rest day/slide day
S	Off	Trans: 45 min. Z2 (at 20 min. insert 20 min. Z4) (QC)	15 min. Z2
S	Off	Opt: 30 min. Z1 (100+ rpm)	2:15 hr. Z1 to Z2
Totals: 7:00+ hr.	1:30 hr.	2:00+ hr.	3:30 hr.

WEEK 15	SWIM	BIKE	RUN
M	Rest day/ slide day	Rest day/slide day	Rest day/slide day
T	#33	Off	45 min. Z2 (at 25 min., insert 15 min. Z4)
W	Off	Trans: 30 min. Z2 (QC)	15 min. Z2
R	#34	45 min. Z2 (at 10 min., insert 3 x 7 min. Z4@3.5 min. spin)	Off
F	Rest day/ slide day	Rest day/slide day	Rest day/slide day
S	Off	Trans: 2:15 hr. Z2 (QC)	15 min. Z2
S	Off	Off	1:15 hr. Z1 to Z2
Totals: 7:30 hr.	1:30 hr.	3:30 hr.	2:30 hr.

WEEK 16	SWIM	BIKE	RUN
M	Rest day/ slide day	Rest day/slide day	Rest day/slide day
T	0.5 hr. easy	Off	45 min. Z1 to Z2 (at 10 min., insert 5 x 1 min. PU@1 min. jog)
W	Off	Trans: 30 min. Z1 to Z2 (QC)	15 min. Z1 to Z2
R	0.5 hr. easy	45 min. Z1 (at 10 min., insert 5 x 1 min. PU @ 1 min. spin)	Off
F	Rest day/ slide day	Rest day/slide day	Rest day/slide day
S	Off	15 min. Z1—easy bike safety check	30 min. Z1—easy (in a.m.)
S	Race!! Half-Iron Distance	Race!! Half-Iron Distance	Race!! Half Iron-Distance
Totals: 4:00+ hr.	1:00 hr. (+R)	1:30 hr. (+Race)	1:30 hr. (+Race)

Guidelines for Adjusting Sixteen-Week Training Programs

In this section we will offer suggestions on how best to make adjustments to the sixteen-week training programs for practice races, missed workouts, and other situations.

Adjusting Training Program for Practice Races

There are up to three optional practice races to include during the three sixteen-week programs. In the following section we present how best to build the three possible races into your sixteen-week training schedule, should you decide that you want to include any or all of them.

Adjusting Training Program for an Open-Water Swim

An open-water swim practice race is beneficial for most triathletes, especially for those who have not raced in open water recently.

The preferable distance is about 1 mile (or about 1.5 km) and it can be substituted for any of the planned swims. If your Half is going to have a wet suit–legal swim, this is an excellent opportunity to become used to swimming in a wet suit if you are not already. Preferably, you will wear the same wet suit for your open-water swim as you plan to wear in your Half.

We don't suggest tapering for this particular training race, but instead just use it as a training session. Since open-water swims are typically on Saturday or Sunday mornings, our suggestion is to simply complete it in the morning before your other bike and/or run training planned for that day and to count it toward any of your planned swim sessions. Any weekend between week four and week fifteen are fine for this practice race, as long as you are at a point where you feel safe and comfortable in the open water.

Adjusting Training Program for a Sprint or Olympic Distance Triathlon

Either a Sprint or Olympic Distance triathlon can serve as a great "dress-rehearsal" for your Half.

The best weeks in the training programs to include a Sprint Triathlon (approximately a 0.5-mile swim, a 15-mile bike, and a 3-mile run) or an Olympic Distance Triathlon (approximately a 1.5K swim, a 40K bike, and a 10K run) tune-up race are weeks ten through fourteen, and it is suggested that you adjust the days around the race as follows:

Friday: 30-minute easy swim and 60 min. Z1 to Z2 run with 5 x 1 min. Easy Pickups @ 1 min. jog).

Saturday: 30-minute Z1 easy run in morning and 30 min. Z1 easy bike safety check anytime later in the day.

Sunday: Sprint or Olympic Distance Race in the morning, then a 2:00-to-3:00 hr. Z1 to Z2 bike session anytime later in the day.

Monday: Complete long run originally planned for Sunday.

Tuesday: Rejoin training schedule as planned, however, do not include Z4 portion of Tuesday's run. Instead, just cover the time of Tuesday's run in Z2.

Adjusting Training Program for a Half Marathon

A Half Marathon can be a beneficial practice race for athletes who do not come from a running background or who have not completed this distance of a road race in a while.

The best weeks in the training program to include a Half Marathon (13.1 miles) are during weeks ten through fourteen, and it is suggested that you just substitute this race in for one of your Sunday long runs. The one suggested adjustment to the schedule is not to include the Z4 Insert in the bike session on the day before the Half Marathon. Otherwise, no other adjustments are needed to the schedule. Just treat it as a fast and fun training run.

It is suggested that if you plan to do both a Half Marathon and a Sprint or Olympic Distance Triathlon that you do not do them on consecutive weekends. Spread them apart by at least two weeks.

Adjusting Training Program for Missed Workouts and other Program Adjustment Tips

See pages 136 and 137 for suggestions on how best to adjust the training programs in this book for missed workouts, plus other great program adjustment tips.

Now that we have presented the three Sixteen-Week Half Iron-Distance Training programs, we will move on to Chapter 12, where we will present our Full Iron-Distance Training Programs.

Training Programs for Full Iron-Distance Triathlons

This chapter includes three detailed twenty/thirty-week Full Iron-Distance (approximately a 2.4-mile swim, 112-mile bike, and 26.2-mile run) training programs. Each program is based on the number of hours an athlete has available to train and level of competitiveness.

We refer to these training programs as "twenty/thirty week" because while the actual program presented covers the twenty weeks before the Iron Distance competition, each program also presents specific recommendations for exactly how best to train and prepare in the ten weeks before the athlete begins the twenty-week program.

The Competitive Program includes approximately 275 total training hours, with an average of about 13.75 hours per week and a maximum week of about twenty hours. The Intermediate Program has about 220 total training hours, with an average of about eleven hours per week and a maximum week of about fourteen hours. The Just-Finish Program tops out at about 165 total training hours, with an average of about 8.25 hours per week and a maximum week of about ten hours. The reader simply selects the program that best fits her goals, competitiveness, level of experience, and available training time.

Each program tells the reader exactly what to do each and every day throughout the twenty-week period. There are none of the complicated formulas or overly general workout descriptions often found in other training books. Having worked with hundreds of female athletes for many years, we know that this is not what athletes want. Athletes want clear direction on exactly what they need to do and when. This is exactly what these programs provide. The programs are designed to be efficient, productive, and enjoyable.

Following is a summary comparison of the three twenty-week programs.

TRAINING PROGRAM	AVERAGE HOURS/WEEK	PEAK HOURS/WEEK	TOTAL HOURS (APPROX.)
Competitive	13.75	20.0	275
Intermediate	11.0	14.0	220
Just-Finish	8.25	10.0	165

Consider the time management techniques presented in Chapter 2 and in the athlete profiles, and conservatively estimate your weekly training time availability. Once you have completed this analysis, simply select the program that best fits you, your goals, your experience level, and your available training time.

Each program provides specific guidance on what to do in the ten weeks prior to starting the twenty-week program. The focus over these ten weeks is on establishing a sound aerobic base and gradually increasing durations in each of the three sports. Following this initial ten-week "base phase" the athlete is ready to begin the twenty-week program. Each twenty-week program has a similar format. All are constructed with two ten-week phases: the "build phase," and "peak training phase."

Abbreviations for Training Programs

See page 110.

Notes to Swim Sessions in Training Programs

See page 111.

Twenty-Week Training Programs

Following are our three twenty-week training programs and full explanations of each, starting with the Twenty-Week Competitive Program.

Competitive Twenty-Week Training Program

The Competitive Program is for the experienced athlete who wants to maximize her potential and has available time to train for an average of about 13.75 hours a week, with several peak weeks of about twenty hours. The total combined training time over the twenty-week period is approximately 275 hours so we also like to refer to this as the "275-hour plan."

Is Your Body Prepared to Begin the Program?

If you have already been training consistently for ten weeks or more and averaging ten hours per week or more in recent weeks, with at least two sessions per week in each of the three sports, then you can skip the base-building phase and begin the twenty-week Iron-Distance program. If you are either starting from scratch or some level less than this, then we suggest a ten-week pre-phase to establish your aerobic base and build up your durations.

Our suggestion is to start with a five- to six-hour training week of two swim sessions totaling one to two hours, three bike sessions totaling about two hours, and three run sessions totaling about two hours. Then, over the ten-week period, gradually increase your total weekly time by about 30 minutes per week, bringing your total hours up to about ten to eleven hours per week.

Suggestions for this ten-week buildup phase:

- Keep all training fully aerobic (heart rates Z1 and Z2).
- Swim sessions should remain at two to three sessions per week and one hour per session.
- Bike sessions should remain at three sessions per week. Two of these sessions should build to 60 minutes and the third should continue to build up to three hours.
- Run sessions should remain at three sessions per week, building to 60 minutes each.

Once you have gradually and safely built up to these levels over a ten-week period, you are ready to begin our twenty-week training program.

Base-Building Phase: Weeks One through Ten

The first ten weeks of the twenty-week program is the build phase. We start at about ten hours and we introduce higher-intensity training in the first week. From there, both our Z4 portions and durations gradually build to a total of about sixteen hours by the tenth week. This amount assumes two swims of about one hour per week, but this program also includes an optional third swim, which adds another hour to these totals. If swimming is your weakest of the three sports, it will be very helpful to include the third swim if possible.

Our longest sessions in the first ten weeks will be a five-hour transition session (Trans: 4:15 hr. Z2 bike [QC] 45 min. Z2 run) and a two-hour Z1 to Z2 run on the last weekend of the tenth week.

The following chart details the ten-week build phase of the Competitive Program:

COMPETITIVE PROGRAM — BUILD PHASE

WEEK 1	SWIM	BIKE	RUN
M	#1—Opt.	Rest day/slide day	Rest day/slide day
T	Off	Off	1:00 hr. Z2 (at 10 min. insert 5 x 1 min. PU @ 1 min. jog)
W	#2	Trans: 45 min. Z2 (QC)	15 min. Z2
R	Off	1:00 hr. Z2 (at 10 min., insert 5 x 1 min. PU @ 1 min. spin)	Off
F	#3	Off	1:00 hr. Z2 (at 45 min. insert 5 x 1 min. PU @ 1 min. jog)
S	Off	2:45 hr. Z2 (at 2:30, insert 5 x 1 min. PU @ 1 min. spin)	Off
S	Off	Off	1:15 hr. Z1 to Z2
Totals: 10:00+ hr.	2:00+ hr.	4:30 hr.	3:30 hr.

WEEK 2	SWIM	BIKE	RUN
M	#4—Opt.	Rest day/slide day	Rest day/slide day
T	Off	Off	1:00 hr. Z2 (at 10 min. insert 8 x 2 min. Z4 @ 1 min. jog)
W	#5	Trans: 45 min. Z2 (QC)	15 min. Z2
R	Off	1:00 hr. Z2 (at 10 min., insert 10 x 2 min. Z4 Hill Repeats @ spin back down)	Off
F	#6	Off	1:00 hr. Z2 (at 45 min., insert 5 min. Z4)
S	Off	2:45 hr. Z2 (at 2:30 hr. insert 5 min. Z4)	Off
S	Off	Off	1:15 hr. Z1 to Z2
Totals: 10:00+ hr.	2:00+ hr.	4:30 hr.	3:30 hr.

WEEK 3	SWIM	BIKE	RUN
M	#7—Opt.	Rest day/slide day	Rest day/slide day
T	Off	Off	1:00 hr. Z2 (at 10 min. insert 7 x 3 min. Z4 @ 1.5 min. jog)
W	#8	Trans: 45 min. Z2 (QC)	15 min. Z2
R	Off	1:00 hr. Z2 (at 10 min., insert 6 x 4 min. Z4 @ 2 min. spin)	Off
F	#9	Off	1:00 hr. Z2 (at 45 min., insert 7.5 min. Z4)
S	Off	Trans: 2:45 hr. Z2 (at 2:30 hr. insert 7.5 min. Z4) (QC)	15 min. Z2
S	Off	30 min. Z1 (100+ rpm)	1:15 hr. Z1 to Z2
Totals: 10:45+ hr.	2:00+ hr.	5:00 hr.	3:45 hr.

COMPETITIVE PROGRAM — BUILD PHASE

WEEK 4	SWIM	BIKE	RUN
M	#10—Opt.	Rest day/slide day	Rest day/slide day
T	Off	Off	1:00 hr. Z2 (at 10 min. insert 6 x 4.5 min. Z4 @ 2 min. jog)
W	#11	Trans: 45 min. Z2 (QC)	15 min. Z2
R	Off	1:00 hr. Z2 (at 10 min., insert 10 x 2.5 min. Z4 Hill Repeats @ spin back down)	Off
F	#12	Off	1:00 hr. Z2 (at 60 min., insert 10 min. Z4)
S	Off	Trans: 3:15 hr. Z2 (at 3:00 hr. insert 10 min. Z4) (QC)	15 min. Z2
S	Off	30 min. Z1 (100+ rpm)	1:30 hr. Z1 to Z2
Totals: 11:30+ hr.	2:00+ hr.	5:30 hr.	4:00 hr.

WEEK 5	SWIM	BIKE	RUN
M	#13—Opt.	Rest day/slide day	Rest day/slide day
T	Off	Off	1:00 hr. Z2 (at 10 min. insert 5 x 6 min. Z4 @ 3 min. jog)
W	#14	Trans: 45 min. Z2 (QC)	15 min. Z2
R	Off	1:15 hr. Z2 (at 10 min., insert 5 x 5 min. Z4 @ 2.5 min. spin)	Off
F	#15	Off	1:00 hr. Z2 (at 40 min., insert 12.5 min. Z4)
S	Off	Trans: 3:30 hr. Z2 (at 3:10 hr. insert 12.5 min. Z4) (QC)	30 min. Z2
S	Off	30 min. Z1 (100+ rpm)	1:30 hr. Z1 to Z2
Totals: 12:15+ hr.	2:00+ hr.	6:00 hr.	4:15 hr.

WEEK 6	SWIM	BIKE	RUN
M	#16—Opt.	Rest day/slide day	Rest day/slide day
T	Off	Off	1:00 hr. Z2 (at 10 min. insert 4 x 7.5 min. Z4 @ 3.5 min. jog)
W	#17	Trans: 45 min. Z2 (QC)	15 min. Z2
R	Off	1:15 hr. Z2 (at 10 min. insert 10 x 3 min. Z4 Hill Repeats @ spin back down)	Off
F	#18	Off	1:15 hr. Z2 (at 55 min., insert 15 min. Z4)
S	Off	Trans: 3:30 hr. Z2 (at 3:10 hr. insert 15 min. Z4) (QC)	30 min. Z2
S	Off	60 min. Z1 (100+ rpm)	1:30 hr. Z1 to Z2
Totals: 13:00+ hr.	2:00+ hr.	6:30 hr.	4:30 hr.

WEEK 7	SWIM	BIKE	RUN
M	#19—Opt.	Rest day/slide day	Rest day/slide day
T	Off	Off	1:00 hr. Z2 (at 10 min., insert 10 x 3 min. Z4 @ 1.5 min. jog)
W	#20	Trans: 45 min. Z2 (QC)	15 min. Z2
R	Off	1:30 hr. Z2 (at 10 min., insert 4 x 7.5 min. Z4 @ 3.5 min. spin)	Off
F	#21	Off	1:15 hr. Z2 (at 55 min., insert 15 min. Z4)
S	Off	Trans: 3:45 hr. Z2 (at 3:25 hr. insert 15 min. Z4) (QC)	30 min. Z2
S	Off	60 min. Z1 (100+ rpm)	1:45 hr. Z1 to Z2
Totals: 13:45+ hr.	2:00+ hr.	7:00 hr.	4:45 hr.

COMPETITIVE PROGRAM — BUILD PHASE

WEEK 8	SWIM	BIKE	RUN
M	#22—Opt.	Rest day/slide day	Rest day/slide day
T	Off	Off	1:00 hr. Z2 (at 10 min. insert, 6 x 4.5 min. Z4 @ 2 min. jog)
W	#23	Trans: 45 min. Z2 (QC)	30 min. Z2
R	Off	1:30 hr. Z2 (at 10 min. insert 8 x 3.5 min. Z4 Hill Repeats @ spin back down)	Off
F	#24	Off	1:15 hr. Z2 (at 55 min. insert 15 min. Z4)
S	Off	Trans: 3:45 hr. Z2 (at 3:25 hr. insert 15 min. Z4) (QC)	45 min. Z2
S		75 min. Z1 (100+ rpm)	1:45 hr. Z1 to Z2
Totals: 14:30+ hr.	2:00+ hr.	7:15 hr.	5:15 hr.

WEEK 9	SWIM	BIKE	RUN
M	#2—Opt.	Rest day/slide day	Rest day/slide day
T	Off	Off	1:15 hr. Z2 (at 10 min. insert 5 x 6 min. Z4 @ 3 min. jog)
W	#1	Trans: 60 min. Z2 (QC)	30 min. Z2
R	Off	1:30 hr. Z2 (at 10 min., insert 6 x 5 min. Z4 @ 2.5 min. spin)	Off
F	#3	Off	1:15 hr. Z2 (at 55 min., insert 15 min. Z4)
S	Off	Trans: 4:00 hr. Z2 (at 3:40 hr. insert 15 min. Z4) (QC)	30 min. Z2
S	Off	75 min. Z1 (100+ rpm)	2:00 hr. Z1 to Z2
Totals: 15:15+ hr.	2:00+ hr.	7:45 hr.	5:30 hr.

WEEK 10	SWIM	BIKE	RUN
M	#5—Opt.	Rest day/slide day	Rest day/slide day
T	Off	Off	1:15 hr. Z2 (at 10 min. insert 4 x 7.5 min. Z4 @ 3.5 min. jog)
W	#4	Trans: 60 min. Z2 (QC)	30 min. Z2
R	Off	1:30 hr. Z2 (at 10 min. insert 15 x 2 min. Z4 Hill Repeats @ spin back down)	Off
F	#6	Off	1:15 hr. Z2 (at 55 min., insert 15 min. Z4)
S	Off	Trans: 4:15 hr. Z2 (at 3:55 hr. insert 15 min. Z3) (QC)	45 min. Z2
S	Off	90 min. Z1 (100+ rpm)	2:00 hr. Z1 to Z2
Totals: 16:00+ hr.	2:00+ hr.	8:15 hr.	5:45 hr.

Swim Sessions for the Competitive Program

Our swims for the Competitive Program will all be approximately 3,000 yards or meters in length, which is a workout distance most athletes can complete within one hour. Our suggestion is that if you need to lengthen the session to last a full hour, simply extend the warm-up and/or cooldown portion as needed. If, however, you find you need to shorten the session to make it fit into an hour, reduce the main sets as needed but keep the warm-up, drills, and cooldown the same.

See page 112 for the numbered swim sessions to be used with this training program.

Peak Training and Taper Phases: Weeks Eleven through Twenty

The second ten weeks (weeks eleven through twenty) of the Competitive Program include both the peak training phase and the taper phase. Our weekly training hours will build to about twenty hours by the fifteenth week and we will maintain 90 minutes of combined weekly cycling and running Z4 training for several of the weeks in this phase.

During the second ten weeks, we will continue to include two swims of about one hour (3,000 yards/meters) each per week, with an optional third swim, which adds another hour to these totals. Again, if swimming is your weakest of the three sports, it will be very helpful to include the third swim if possible.

Our longest sessions in the second ten weeks will be seven-hour transition sessions and three-hour long runs.

In the twelfth week we will have a Half Iron-Distance tune-up race. While we should race this event to the best of our ability, our primary purpose is to use this opportunity to practice all of our race-day routines and logistics. This includes pre-race, race, and post-race fueling and hydration, race equipment, and race clothing. We want to test everything out just like we plan to do it for our actual Iron-Distance triathlon. We will identify any elements that we need to adjust prior to the big day, and completing this Half Iron-Distance race will provide us with extra confidence and experience as we head into our final eight weeks of preparation.

With three weeks to go before our Iron-Distance race, we will transition into our crisp taper phase to have us rested, sharp, and race-ready. Our durations and higher-intensity training will gradually decrease. Within the final nine days before our race, we will not have any training intensities higher than Z2. At this point the hay is in the barn and it is time to taper smart and become physically and mentally energized.

Following is the ten-week peak training and taper phase of the Competitive Program.

COMPETITIVE PROGRAM — PEAK TRAINING AND TAPER PHASES

WEEK 11	SWIM	BIKE	RUN
M	#8—Opt.	Rest day/slide day	Rest day/slide day
T	Off	Off	1:15 hr. Z2 (at 10 min. insert, 10 x 3 min. Z4 @ 1.5 min. jog)
W	#7	Trans: 60 min. Z2 (QC)	30 min. Z2
R	Off	1:30 hr. Z2 (at 10 min., insert 4 x 7.5 min. Z4 @ 3.5 min. spin)	Off
F	#9	Off	1:15 hr. Z2 (at 60 min. insert 10 min. Z4)
S	Off	Trans: 2:30 hr. Z2 (QC)	30 min. Z2
S	Off	30 min. Z1 (100+ rpm)	60 hr. Z1 to Z2
Totals: 12:00+ hr.	2:00+ hr.	5:30 hr.	4:30 hr.

WEEK 12	SWIM	BIKE	RUN
M	Off	Rest day/slide day	Rest day/slide day
T	Off	Off	45 min. Z1 to Z2 (at 10 min. insert 5 x 1 min. PU @1 min. jog)
W	0.5 hr. easy	Trans: 45 min. Z1 to Z2 (QC)	15 min. Z1 to Z2
R	Off	60 min. Z1 (at 10 min. insert 5 x 1 min. PU @ 1 min. spin)	Off
F	0.5 hr. easy	Off	40 min. Z1 (at 10 min., insert 5 x 1 min. PU @ 1 min. jog)
S	Off	15 min. Z1—easy bike safety check	20 min. Z1—easy (in a.m.)
S	Race!!	Race!! Half Iron-Distance	Race!! Half Iron-Distance
Totals: 5:00+ hr.	1:00 hr. (+R)	2:00 hr. (+Race)	2:00 hr. (+Race)

COMPETITIVE PROGRAM — PEAK TRAINING AND TAPER PHASES

WEEK 13	SWIM	BIKE	RUN
M	#11—Opt.	Rest day/slide day	Rest day/slide day
T	Off	Off	60 min. Z1—easy
W	#10	Trans: 1:15 hr. Z2 (QC)	30 min. Z1 to Z2
R	Off	1:30 hr. Z2	Off
F	#12	Off	1:15 hr. Z2
S	Off	Trans: 5:00 hr. Z2 (QC)	45 min. Z2
S	Off	90 min. Z1 (100+ rpm)	3:00 hr. Z1 to Z2
Totals: 17:45+ hr.	2:00+ hr.	9:15 hr.	6:30 hr.

WEEK 14	SWIM	BIKE	RUN
M	#14—Opt.	Rest day/slide day	Rest day/slide day
T	Off	Off	1:15 hr. Z2 (at 10 min. insert 6 x 4.5 min. Z4 @ 2 min. jog)
W	#13	Trans: 1:30 hr. Z2 (QC)	30 min. Z2
R	Off	1:45 hr. Z2 (at 10 min., insert 12 x 2.5 min. Z4 Hill Repeats @ spin back down)	Off
F	#15	Off	1:15 hr. Z2 (at 55 min., insert 15 min. Z4)
S	Off	Trans: 6:00 hr. Z2 (at 5:40 hr. insert 15 min. Z4) (QC)	60 min. Z2
S	Off	90 min. Z1 (100+ rpm)	2:30 hr. Z1 to Z2
Totals: 19:15+ hr.	2:00+ hr.	10:45 hr.	6:30 hr.

WEEK 15	SWIM	BIKE	RUN
M	#17—Opt.	Rest day/slide day	Rest day/slide day
T	Off	Off	1:15 hr. Z2 (at 10 min. insert 5 x 6 min. Z4 @ 3 min. jog)
W	#16	Trans: 1:30 hr. Z2 (QC)	30 min. Z2
R	Off	2:00 hr. Z2 (at 10 min., insert 6 x 5 min. Z4 @ 2.5 min. spin)	Off
F	#18	Off	1:30 hr. Z2 (at 1:10, insert 15 min. Z4)
S	Off	Trans: 6:00 hr. Z2 (at 5:40 hr. insert 15 min. Z4) (QC)	60 min. Z2
S	Off	90 min. Z1 (100+ rpm)	3:00 hr. Z1 to Z2
Totals: 20:15+ hr.	2:00+ hr.	11:00 hr.	7:15 hr.

WEEK 16	SWIM	BIKE	RUN
M	#20—Opt.	Rest day/slide day	Rest day/slide day
T	Off	Off	1:15 hr. Z2 (at 10 min. insert 4 x 7.5 min. Z4 @ 3.5 min. jog)
W	#19	Trans: 1:30 hr. Z2 (QC)	30 min. Z2
R	Off	2:00 hr. Z2 (at 10 min. insert 10 x 3 min. Z4 Hill Repeats @ spin back down)	Off
F	#21	Off	1:30 hr. Z2 (at 1:10, insert 15 min. Z4)
S	Off	Trans: 6:00 hr. Z2 (at 5:40 hr. insert 15 min. Z4) (QC)	60 min. Z2
S	Off	90 min. Z1 (100+ rpm)	2:30 hr. Z1 to Z2
Totals: 19:45+ hr.	2:00+ hr.	11:00 hr.	6:45 hr.

COMPETITIVE PROGRAM — PEAK TRAINING AND TAPER PHASES

WEEK 17	SWIM	BIKE	RUN
M	#23—Opt.	Rest day/slide day	Rest day/slide day
T	Off	Off	1:15 hr. Z2 (at 10 min. insert 1 x 10 min. Z4 @ 5 min. jog, then 10 x 2 min. Z4 @ 1 min. jog)
W	#22	Trans: 1:30 hr. Z2 (QC)	30 min. Z2
R	Off	2:00 hr. Z2 (at 10 min., insert 4 x 7.5 min. Z4 @ 3.5 min. spin)	Off
F	#24	Off	1:30 hr. Z2 (at 1:10, insert 15 min. Z4)
S	Off	Trans: 6:00 hr. Z2 (at 5:40 hr. insert 15 min. Z4) (QC)	60 min. Z2
S	Off	90 min. Z1 (100+ rpm)	3:00 hr. Z1 to Z2
Totals: 20:15+ hr.	2:00+ hr.	11:00 hr.	7:15 hr.

WEEK 18	SWIM	BIKE	RUN
M	#1—Opt.	Rest day/slide day	Rest day/slide day
T	Off	Off	1:15 hr. Z2 (at 10 min. insert 3 x 6 min. Z4 @ 3 min. jog)
W	#2	Trans: 1:15 hr. Z2 (QC)	30 min. Z2
R	Off	1:45 hr. Z2 (at 10 min., insert 2 x 10 min. Z4 @ 5 min. spin)	Off
F	#3	Off	1:15 hr. Z2 (at 55 min., insert 12.5 min. Z4)
S	Off	Trans: 4:15 hr. Z2 (at 4:00 hr. insert 10 min. Z4) (QC)	45 min. Z2
S		75 min. Z1 (100+ rpm)	2:15 hr. Z1 to Z2
Totals: 16:30+ hr.	2:00+ hr.	8:30 hr.	6:00 hr.

WEEK 19	SWIM	BIKE	RUN
M	#4—Opt.	Rest day/slide day	Rest day/slide day
T	Off	Off	60 min. Z2 (at 10 min. insert 4 x 3 min. Z4 @ 1.5 min. jog)
W	#5	Trans: 60 min. Z2 (QC)	30 min. Z2
R	Off	1:30 hr. Z2 (at 1:15 hr., insert 10 min. Z4)	Off
F	#6	Off	1:15 hr. Z2 (at 60 min., insert 10 min. Z4)
S	Off	Trans: 2:30 hr. Z2 (QC)	30 min. Z2
S	Off	30 min. Z1 (100+ rpm)	1:15 hr. Z1 to Z2
Totals: 12:00+ hr.	2:00+ hr.	5:30 hr.	4:30 hr.

WEEK 20	SWIM	BIKE	RUN
M	Off	Rest day/slide day	Rest day/slide day
T	Off	Off	45 min. Z1 to Z2 (at 10 min. insert 5 x 1 min. PU @ 1 min. jog)
W	0.5 hr. easy	Trans: 45 min. Z1 to Z2 (QC)	15 min. Z1 to Z2
R	Off	60 min. Z1 (at 10 min. insert 5 x 1 min. PU @ 1 min. spin)	Off
F	0.5 hr. easy	Off	40 min. Z1 (at 10 min., insert 5 x 1 min. PU @ 1 min. jog)
S	Off	15 min. Z1—easy bike safety check	20 min. Z1—easy (in a.m.)
S	Race!!	Race!! Full Iron-Distance	Race!! Full Iron-Distance
Totals: 5:00+ hr.	1:00 hr. (+R)	2:00 hr. (+Race)	2:00 hr. (+Race)

Intermediate Twenty-Week Training Program

What if the Competitive Program sounds like too much, but you feel that you can squeeze out a little more weekly training time than is required for the Just-Finish Program? What if you don't dream of making it to the awards podium, but you would like to do more than just finish?

The Intermediate Program is a compromise in time commitment between the Competitive Program and the Just-Finish Program. It requires an average of about eleven hours a week, with several peak weeks of about fifteen hours. The total combined training time over the twenty-week period is approximately 220 hours, so we also like to refer to this as the "220-hour plan."

Is Your Body Prepared to Begin the Twenty-Week Program?

If you have already been training consistently for ten weeks or more and averaging eight hours per week or more in recent weeks, with at least two sessions per week in each of the three sports, then you can skip the base-building phase and begin the twenty-week Iron-Distance program. If you are either starting from scratch or some level less than this, then we suggest a ten-week pre-phase to establish your aerobic base and build up your durations.

Our suggestion is to start with a four- to five-hour training week of two swim sessions totaling one to two hours, three bike sessions totaling about two hours, and three run sessions totaling about two hours. Then, over the ten-week period, gradually increase your total weekly time by about 30 minutes per week, bringing your total hours up to about seven to eight hours per week.

Suggestions for this ten-week build-up phase:

- Keep all training fully aerobic (heart rates Z1 and Z2).
- Swim sessions should remain at two to three sessions per week and one hour per session.
- Bike sessions should remain at three sessions per week. Two of these sessions should build to 60 minutes and the third should continue to build up to three hours.
- Run sessions should remain at three sessions per week, building to 60 minutes each.

Once you have gradually and safely built up to these levels over a ten-week period, you are ready to begin our twenty-week training program.

Base Building Phase: Weeks One through Ten

The first ten weeks of the twenty-week program is the build phase. We start at nine and three-quarters hours and we introduce higher-intensity training in the first week. From there, both our Z4 portions and durations gradually build to a total of about twelve hours by the tenth week. This amount assumes two swims of about one hour per week, but this program also includes an optional third swim, which adds another hour to these totals. If swimming is your weakest of the three sports, it will be very helpful to include the third swim if possible.

Our longest sessions in the first ten weeks will be a four-hour bike session and a two-hour run on the last weekend of the tenth week.

The following chart details the ten-week build phase of the Intermediate Program.

INTERMEDIATE PROGRAM — BASE-BUILDING PHASE

WEEK 1	SWIM	BIKE	RUN
M	#1—Opt.	Rest day/slide day	Rest day/slide day
T	Off	Off	1:00 hr. Z2 (at 10 min. insert 5 x 1 min. PU @ 1 min. jog)
W	#2	Trans: 45 min. Z2 (QC)	15 min. Z2
R	Off	60 min. Z2 (at 10 min. insert 5 x 1 min. PU @ 1 min. spin)	Off
F	#3	Off	1:00 hr. Z2 (at 45 min. insert 5 min. Z4)
S	Off	2:30 hr. Z2 (at 2:15 hr. insert 5 min. Z4)	Off
S	Off	Off	1:15 hr. Z1 to Z2
Totals: 9:45+ hr.	2:00+ hr.	4:15 hr.	3:30 hr.

INTERMEDIATE PROGRAM — BASE-BUILDING PHASE

WEEK 2	SWIM	BIKE	RUN
M	#4—Opt.	Rest day/slide day	Rest day/slide day
T	Off	Off	45 min. Z2 (at 10 min. insert 6 x 2 min. Z4 @ 1 min. jog)
W	#5	Trans: 45 min. Z2 (QC)	15 min. Z2
R	Off	60 min. Z2 (at 10 min. insert 7 x 2 min. Z4 Hill Repeats @ spin back down)	Off
F	#6	Off	1:00 hr. Z2 (at 45 min., 5 min. Z4)
S	Off	3:00 hr. Z2 (at 2:45 hr. insert 5 min. Z4)	Off
S	Off	Off	1:15 hr. Z1 to Z2
Totals: 10:00+ hr.	2:00+ hr.	4:45 hr.	3:15 hr.

WEEK 3	SWIM	BIKE	RUN
M	#7—Opt.	Rest day/slide day	Rest day/slide day
T	Off	Off	45 min. Z2 (at 10 min. insert 5 x 3 min. Z4 @ 1.5 min. jog)
W	#8	Trans: 45 min. Z2 (QC)	15 min. Z2
R	Off	60 min. Z2 (at 10 min., insert 4 x 4 min. Z4 @ 2 min. spin)	Off
F	#9	Off	1:00 hr. Z2 (at 45 min., insert 7.5 min. Z4)
S	Off	3:00 hr. Z2 (at 2:45 hr. insert 7.5 min. Z4)	Off
S		Off	1:15 hr. Z1 to Z2
Totals: 10:00+ hr.	2:00+ hr.	4:45 hr.	3:15 hr.

WEEK 4	SWIM	BIKE	RUN
M	#10—Opt.	Rest day/slide day	Rest day/slide day
T	Off	Off	1:00 hr. Z2 (at 10 min. insert 4 x 4.5 min. Z4 @ 2 min. jog)
W	#11	Trans: 45 min. Z2 (QC)	15 min. Z2
R	Off	60 min. Z2 (at 10 min. insert 8 x 2.5 min. Z4 Hill Repeats @ spin back down)	Off
F	#12	Off	1:00 hr. Z2 (at 45 min. insert 10 min. Z4)
S	Off	3:30 hr. Z2 (at 3:15 hr. insert 10 min. Z4)	Off
S	Off	Off	1:15 hr. Z1 to Z2
Totals: 10:45+ hr.	2:00+ hr.	5:15 hr.	3:30 hr.

WEEK 5	SWIM	BIKE	RUN
M	#13—Opt.	Rest day/slide day	Rest day/slide day
T	Off	Off	1:00 hr. Z2 (at 10 min. insert 4 x 6 min. Z4 @ 3 min. jog)
W	#14	Trans: 45 min. Z2 (QC)	15 min. Z2
R	Off	60 min. Z2 (at 10 min. insert 4 x 5 min. Z4 @ 2.5 min. spin)	Off
F	#15	Off	1:00 hr. Z2 (at 40 min., insert 12.5 min. Z4)
S	Off	4:00 hr. Z2 (at 3:40 hr. insert 12.5 min. Z4)	Off
S	Off	Off	1:30 hr. Z1 to Z2
Totals: 11:30+ hr.	2:00+ hr.	5:45 hr.	3:45 hr.

INTERMEDIATE PROGRAM — BASE-BUILDING PHASE

WEEK 6	SWIM	BIKE	RUN
M	#16—Opt.	Rest day/slide day	Rest day/slide day
T	Off	Off	60 min. Z2 (at 10 min. insert 3 x 7.5 min. Z4 @ 3.5 min. jog)
W	#17	Trans: 45 min. Z2 (QC)	15 min. Z2
R	Off	60 min. Z2 (at 10 min. insert 7 x 3 min. Z4 Hill Repeats @ spin back down)	Off
F	#18	Off	1:00 hr. Z2 (at 40 min., insert 15 min. Z4)
S	Off	3:00 hr. Z2 (at 2:40 hr. insert 15 min. Z4)	Off
S	Off	Off	1:30 hr. Z1 to Z2
Totals: 10:30+ hr.	2:00+ hr.	4:45 hr.	3:45 hr.

WEEK 7	SWIM	BIKE	RUN
M	#19—Opt.	Rest day/slide day	Rest day/slide day
T	Off	Off	1:00 hr. Z2 (at 10 min. insert 8 x 3 min. Z4 @ 1.5 min. jog)
W	#20	Trans: 45 min. Z2 (QC)	15 min. Z2
R	Off	60 min. Z2 (at 10 min. insert 3 x 7.5 min. Z4 @ 3.5 min. spin)	Off
F	#21	Off	1:00 hr. Z2 (at 40 min., insert 15 min. Z4)
S	Off	3:30 hr. Z2 (at 3:10 hr. insert 15 min. Z4)	Off
S	Off	Off	1:15 hr. Z1 to Z2
Totals: 10:45+ hr.	2:00+ hr.	5:15 hr.	3:30 hr.

WEEK 8	SWIM	BIKE	RUN
M	#22—Opt.	Rest day/slide day	Rest day/slide day
T	Off	Off	1:00 hr. Z2 (at 10 min. insert 5 x 4.5 min. Z4 @ 2 min. jog)
W	#23	Trans: 45 min. Z2 (QC)	15 min. Z2
R	Off	60 min. Z2 (at 10 min. insert 6 x 3.5 min. Z4 Hill Repeats @ spin back down)	Off
F	#24	Off	1:00 hr. Z2 (at 40 min., insert 15 min. Z4)
S	Off	3:30 hr. Z2 (at 3:10 hr. insert 15 min. Z4)	Off
S	Off	Off	1:30 hr. Z1 to Z2
Totals: 11:00+ hr.	2:00+ hr.	5:15 hr.	3:45 hr.

WEEK 9	SWIM	BIKE	RUN
M	#2—Opt.	Rest day/slide day	Rest day/slide day
T	Off	Off	1:00 hr. Z2 (at 10 min. insert 4 x 6 min. Z4 @ 3 min. jog)
W	#1	Trans: 45 min. Z2 (QC)	15 min. Z2
R	Off	60 min. Z2 (at 10 min. insert 4 x 5 min. Z4 @ 2.5 spin)	Off
F	#3	Off	1:00 hr. Z2 (at 40 min., insert 15 min. Z4)
S	Off	4:00 hr. Z2 (at 3:40 hr. insert 15 min. Z4)	Off
S	Off	Off	1:30 hr. Z1 to Z2
Totals: 11:30+ hr.	2:00+ hr.	5:45 hr.	3:45 hr.

INTERMEDIATE PROGRAM — BASE-BUILDING PHASE

WEEK 10	SWIM	BIKE	RUN
M	#5—Opt.	Rest day/slide day	Rest day/slide day
T	Off	Off	1:00 hr. Z2 (at 10 min. insert 3 x 7.5 min. Z4 @ 3.5 min. jog)
W	#4	Trans: 45 min. Z2 (QC)	15 min. Z2
R	Off	60 min. Z2 (at 10 min. insert 10 x 2 min. Z4 Hill Repeats @ spin back down)	Off
F	#6	Off	1:00 hr. Z2 (at 40 min., insert 15 min. Z4)
S	Off	4:00 hr. Z2 (at 3:40 hr. insert 15 min. Z4)	Off
S	Off	Off	2:00 hr. Z1 to Z2
Totals: 12:00+ hr.	2:00+ hr.	5:45 hr.	4:15 hr.

Swim Sessions for the Intermediate Program

Our swims for the Intermediate Program will be approximately 3,000 yards or meters in length, which is a workout distance most athletes can complete within one hour. Our suggestion is that if you need to lengthen the session to last a full hour, simply extend the warm-up and/or cooldown portions as needed. If, however, you find you need to shorten the session to make it fit into an hour, reduce the main sets as needed but keep the warm-up, drills, and cooldown the same.

See page 112 for the numbered swim sessions to be used with this training program.

Peak Training and Taper Phases: Weeks Eleven through Twenty

The second ten weeks (weeks eleven through twenty) of the Intermediate Program include both the peak training phase and the taper phase. Our weekly training hours will build to about fourteen hours by the fifteenth week and we will maintain about 70 to 75 minutes of combined weekly cycling and running Z4 training for several of the weeks in this phase.

During the second ten weeks, we will continue to include two swims of about one hour (3,000 yards/meters) each per week, with an optional third swim, which adds another hour to these totals. Again, if swimming is your weakest of the three sports, it will be very helpful to include the third swim if possible.

Our longest sessions in the second ten weeks will be a couple of 5.5-hour bike sessions and a couple of three-hour long runs.

In the twelfth week we will have a Half Iron-Distance tune-up race. While we should race this event to the best of our ability, our primary purpose is to use this opportunity to practice all of our race-day routines and logistics. This includes pre-race, race, and post-race fueling and hydration, race equipment, and race clothing. We want to test everything out just like we plan to do it for our actual Iron-Distance triathlon. We will identify any elements that we need to adjust prior to the big day, and completing this Half Iron-Distance race will provide us with extra confidence and experience as we head into our final eight weeks of preparation.

With three weeks to go before our Iron-Distance race, we will transition into our crisp taper phase to have us rested, sharp, and race-ready. Our durations and higher-intensity training will gradually decrease. Within the final nine days before our race, we will not have any training intensities higher than Z2. At this point the hay is in the barn and it is time to taper smart and become physically and mentally energized.

Following is the ten-week peak training phase and taper phase of the Intermediate Program.

INTERMEDIATE PROGRAM — PEAK TRAINING AND TAPER PHASES

WEEK 11	SWIM	BIKE	RUN
M	#8—Opt.	Rest day/slide day	Rest day/slide day
T	Off	Off	1:00 hr. Z2 (at 10 min. insert 8 x 3 min. Z4 @ 1.5 min. jog)
W	#7	Trans: 45 min. Z2 (QC)	15 min. Z2
R	Off	60 min. Z2 (at 10 min., insert 3 x 7.5 min. Z4 @ 3.5 min. spin)	Off
F	#9	Off	1:00 hr. Z2 (at 45 min., insert 10 min. Z4)
S	Off	4:00 hr. Z2	Off
S	Off	Off	1:45 hr. Z1 to Z2
Totals: 11:45+ hr.	2:00+ hr.	5:45 hr.	4:00 hr.
WEEK 12	**SWIM**	**BIKE**	**RUN**
M	Off	Rest day/slide day	Rest day/slide day
T	Off	Off	45 min. Z1 to Z2 (at 10 min., insert 5 x 1 min. PU @ 1 min. jog)
W	0.5 hr. easy	Trans: 45 min. Z1 to Z2 (QC)	15 min. Z1 to Z2
R	Off	60 min. Z1 (at 10 min., insert 5 x 1 min. PU @ 1 min. spin)	Off
F	0.5 hr. easy	Off	40 min. Z1 (at 10 min., insert 5 x 1 min. PU @ 1 min. jog)
S	Off	15 min. Z1—easy bike safety check	20 min. Z1—easy (in a.m.)
S	Race!!	Race!! Half Iron-Distance	Race!! Half Iron-Distance
Totals: 5:00+ hr.	1:00+ hr.	2:00 hr. (+Race)	2:00 hr. (+Race)

WEEK 13	SWIM	BIKE	RUN
M	#11—Opt.	Rest day/slide day	Rest day/slide day
T	Off	Off	60 min. Z1-easy
W	#10	Trans: 45 min. Z2 (QC)	15 min. Z2
R	Off	60 min. Z2	Off
F	#12	Off	60 min. Z2
S	Off	5:00 hr. Z2	Off
S	Off	Off	2:00 hr. Z1 to Z2
Totals: 13:00+ hr.	2:00+ hr.	6:45 hr.	4:15 hr.

WEEK 14	SWIM	BIKE	RUN
M	#14—Opt.	Rest day/slide day	Rest day/slide day
T	Off	Off	60 min. Z2 (at 10 min., insert 5 x 4.5 min. Z4 @ 2 min. jog)
W	#13	Trans: 45 min. Z2 (QC)	15 min. Z2
R	Off	60 min. Z2 (at 10 min., insert 9 x 2.5 min. Z4 Hill Repeats @ spin back down)	Off
F	#15	Off	1:00 hr. Z2 (at 40 min., insert 15 min. Z4)
S	Off	5:00 hr. Z2 (at 4:40 hr. insert 15 min. Z4)	Off
S	Off	Off	2:15 hr. Z1 to Z2
Totals: 13:15+ hr.	2:00+ hr.	6:45 hr.	4:30 hr.

INTERMEDIATE PROGRAM — PEAK TRAINING AND TAPER PHASES

WEEK 15	SWIM	BIKE	RUN
M	#17—Opt.	Rest day/slide day	Rest day/slide day
T	Off	Off	1:00 hr. Z2 (at 10 min. insert 4 x 6 min. Z4 @ 3 min. jog)
W	#16	Trans: 45 min. Z2 (QC)	15 min. Z2
R	Off	60 min. Z2 (at 10 min., insert 4 x 5 min. Z4 @ 2.5 min. spin)	Off
F	#18	Off	1:00 hr. Z2 (at 40 min., insert 15 min. Z4)
S	Off	5:30 hr. Z2 (at 5:10 hr. insert 15 min. Z4)	Off
S	Off	Off	2:30 hr. Z1 to Z2
Totals: 14:00+ hr.	2:00+ hr.	7:15 hr.	4:45 hr.

WEEK 16	SWIM	BIKE	RUN
M	#20—Opt.	Rest day/slide day	Rest day/slide day
T	Off	Off	60 min. Z2 (at 10 min., insert 3 x 7.5 min. Z4 @ 3.5 min. jog)
W	#19	Trans: 45 min. Z2 (QC)	15 min. Z2
R	Off	60 min. Z2 (at 10 min., insert 7 x 3 min. Z4 Hill Repeats @ spin back down)	Off
F	#21	Off	1:00 hr. Z2 (at 40 min., insert 15 min. Z4)
S	Off	5:15 hr. Z2 (at 4:55 hr. insert 15 min. Z4)	Off
S	Off	Off	2:45 hr. Z1 to Z2
Totals: 14:00+ hr.	2:00+ hr.	7:00 hr.	5:00 hr.

WEEK 17	SWIM	BIKE	RUN
M	#23—Opt.	Rest day/slide day	Rest day/slide day
T	Off	Off	1:00 hr. Z2 (at 10 min. insert 1 x 10 min. Z4 @ 5 min. jog, the 6 x 2 min. Z4 @ 1 min. jog)
W	#22	Trans: 45 min. Z2 (QC)	15 min. Z2
R	Off	60 min. Z2 (at 10 min., insert 3 x 7.5 min. Z4 @ 3.5 min. spin)	Off
F	#24	Off	1:00 hr. Z2 (at 40 min., insert 15 min. Z4)
S	Off	5:00 hr. Z2 (at 4:40 hr. insert 15 min. Z4)	Off
S	Off	Off	3:00 hr. Z1 to Z2
Totals: 14:00+ hr.	2:00+ hr.	6:45 hr.	5:15 hr.

WEEK 18	SWIM	BIKE	RUN
M	#1—Opt.	Rest day/slide day	Rest day/slide day
T	Off	Off	45 min. Z2 (at 10 min. insert 3 x 6 min. Z4 @ 3 min. jog)
W	#2	Trans: 45 min. Z2 (QC)	15 min. Z2
R	Off	60 min. Z2 (at 10 min. insert 2 x 10 min. Z4 @ 5 min. spin)	Off
F	#3	Off	1:00 hr. Z2 (at 40 min., insert 12.5 min. Z4)
S	Off	4:00 hr. Z2 (at 3:45 hr. insert 10 min. Z4)	Off
S	Off	Off	2:00 hr. Z1 to Z2
Totals: 11:45+ hr.	2:00+ hr.	5:45 hr.	4:00 hr.

INTERMEDIATE PROGRAM — PEAK TRAINING AND TAPER PHASES

WEEK 19	SWIM	BIKE	RUN
M	#4—Opt.	Rest day/slide day	Rest day/slide day
T	Off	Off	45 min. Z2 (at 10 min. insert 4 x 3 min. Z4 @ 1.5 min. jog)
W	#5	Trans: 45 min. Z2 (QC)	15 min. Z2
R	Off	60 min. Z2 (at 45 min., insert 10 min. Z4)	Off
F	#6	Off	1:00 hr. Z2 (at 45 min., insert 10 min. Z4)
S	Off	2:00 hr. Z2	Off
S	Off	Off	1:15 hr. Z1 to Z2
Totals: 9:00+ hr.	2:00+ hr.	3:45 hr.	3:15 hr.

WEEK 20	SWIM	BIKE	RUN
M	Off	Rest day/slide day	Rest day/slide day
T	Off	Off	45 min. Z1 to Z2 (at 10 min., insert 5 x 1 min. PU @ 1 min. jog)
W	0.5 hr. easy	Trans: 45 min. Z1 to Z2 (QC)	15 min. Z1 to Z2
R	Off	60 min. Z1 (at 10 min., insert 5 x 1 min. PU @ 1 min. spin)	Off
F	0.5 hr. easy	Off	40 min. Z1 (at 10 min., insert 5 x 1 min. PU @ 1 min. jog)
S	Off	15 min. Z1—easy bike safety check	20 min. Z1—easy (in a.m.)
S	Race!! Iron-Distance	Race!! Iron-Distance	Race!! Iron-Distance
Totals: 5:00+ hr.	1:00 hr. (+R)	2:00 hr. (+Race)	2:00 hr. (+Race)

Just-Finish Twenty-Week Training Program

The Just-Finish Program is for the athlete who has limited time available to train but would like to be able to complete the Iron-Distance Triathlon safely, in good health, and in good spirits. The Just-Finish Program athlete needs to have available training time of only about 8.5 hours a week, with several peak weeks of about ten hours. The total combined training time over the twenty-week period is approximately 165 hours so we also like to refer to this as the "165-hour plan."

Is Your Body Prepared to Begin the Twenty-Week Program?

If you have already been training consistently for ten weeks or more and averaging six hours per week or more in recent weeks, with at least two sessions per week in each of the three sports, then you can skip the base-building phase and begin the twenty-week Iron-Distance program. If you are either starting from scratch or some level less than this, then we suggest a ten-week pre-phase to establish your aerobic base and build up your durations.

Our suggestion is to start with about three hours of training per week of two swim sessions totaling about one hour, two bike sessions totaling about one hour, and two run sessions totaling about one hour. Then, over the ten-week period, gradually increase your total weekly time by about 15 to 30 minutes per week, bringing your total hours up to about five to six hours per week.

Suggestions for this 10-week build-up phase:

- Keep all training fully aerobic (heart rates Z1 and Z2).
- Swim sessions should remain at two sessions per week, gradually building up to about one hour each.
- Bike sessions should remain at two sessions per week, gradually building up to about one hour each.
- Run sessions should remain at two sessions per week, gradually building up to about one hour each.

Once you have gradually and safely built up to these levels over a ten-week period, you are ready to begin our twenty-week training program.

Base-Building Phase: Weeks One through Ten

The first ten weeks of the twenty-week program is the build phase. We start at about seven hours and then we introduce higher-intensity training in the second week. Our longest sessions in the first ten weeks will be a three-hour bike session and a two-hour run by the last weekend of the tenth week.

The following chart details the ten-week build phase of the Just-Finish Program.

JUST-FINISH PROGRAM — BASE-BUILDING PHASE

WEEK 1	SWIM	BIKE	RUN
M	Rest day/ slide day	Rest day/slide day	Rest day/slide day
T	#25	Off	45 min. Z2 (at 30 min. insert 5 x 1 min. PU @ 1 min. jog)
W	Off	Trans: 30 min. Z2 (QC)	15 min. Z2
R	Off	60 min. Z2 (at 10 min. insert 5 x 1 min. PU @ 1 min. spin)	Off
F	#26	Off	Off
S	Off	2:00 hr. Z2	Off
S	Off	Off	1:00 hr. Z1 to Z2
Totals: 7:00 hr.	1:30 hr.	3:30 hr.	2:00 hr.

WEEK 2	SWIM	BIKE	RUN
M	Rest day/ slide day	Rest day/slide day	Rest day/slide day
T	#27	Off	45 min. Z2 (at 30 min. insert 5 min. Z4)
W	Off	Trans: 30 min. Z2 (QC)	15 min. Z2
R	Off	60 min. Z2 (at 45 min. insert 5 min. Z4)	Off
F	#28	Off	Off
S	Off	2:00 hr. Z2	Off
S	Off	Off	1:15 hr. Z1 to Z2
Totals: 7:15 hr.	1:30 hr.	3:30 hr.	2:15 hr.

WEEK 3	SWIM	BIKE	RUN
M	Rest day/ slide day	Rest day/slide day	Rest day/slide day
T	#29	Off	45 min. Z2 (at 30 min. insert 7.5 min. Z4)
W	Off	Trans: 30 min. Z2 (QC)	15 min. Z2
R	Off	60 min. Z2 (at 45 min. insert 7.5 min. Z4)	Off
F	#30	Off	Off
S	Off	2:15 hr. Z2	Off
S	Off	Off	1:30 hr. Z1 to Z2
Totals: 7:45 hr.	1:30 hr.	3:45 hr.	2:30 hr.

JUST FINISH PROGRAM — BASE-BUILDING PHASE

WEEK 4	SWIM	BIKE	RUN
M	Rest day/ slide day	Rest day/slide day	Rest day/slide day
T	#31	Off	45 min. Z2 (at 30 min. insert 10 min. Z4)
W	Off	Trans: 30 min. Z2 (QC)	15 min. Z2
R	Off	60 min. Z2 (at 45 min. insert 10 min. Z4)	Off
F	#32	Off	Off
S	Off	2:30 hr. Z2	Off
S	Off	Off	1:30 hr. Z1 to Z2
Totals: 8:00 hr.	1:30 hr.	4:00 hr.	2:30 hr.

WEEK 5	SWIM	BIKE	RUN
M	Rest day/ slide day	Rest day/slide day	Rest day/slide day
T	#33	Off	45 min. Z2 (at 25 min. insert 12.5 min. Z4)
W	Off	Trans: 30 min. Z2 (QC)	15 min. Z2
R	Off	60 min. Z2 (at 40 min. insert 12.5 min. Z4)	Off
F	#34	Off	Off
S	Off	2:30 hr. Z2	Off
S	Off	Off	1:30 hr. Z1 to Z2
Totals: 8:00 hr.	1:30 hr.	4:00 hr.	2:30 hr.

WEEK 6	SWIM	BIKE	RUN
M	Rest day/ slide day	Rest day/slide day	Rest day/slide day
T	#35	Off	45 min. Z2 (at 25 min. insert 15 min. Z4)
W	Off	Trans: 30 min. Z2 (QC)	15 min. Z2
R	Off	60 min. Z2 (at 40 min. insert 15 min. Z4)	Off
F	#36	Off	Off
S	Off	2:30 hr. Z2	Off
S	Off	Off	1:30 hr. Z1 to Z2
Totals: 8:00 hr.	1:30 hr.	4:00 hr.	2:30 hr.

WEEK 7	SWIM	BIKE	RUN
M	Rest day/ slide day	Rest day/slide day	Rest day/slide day
T	#37	Off	1:00 hr. Z2 (at 40 min. insert 15 min. Z4)
W	Off	Trans: 30 min. Z2 (QC)	15 min. Z2
R	#38	60 min. Z2 (at 40 min. insert 15 min. Z4)	Off
F	Off	Off	Off
S	Off	2:30 hr. Z2	Off
S	Off	Off	1:30 hr. Z1 to Z2
Totals: 8:15 hr.	1:30 hr.	4:00 hr.	2:45 hr.

JUST FINISH PROGRAM — BASE-BUILDING PHASE

WEEK 8	SWIM	BIKE	RUN
M	Rest day/ slide day	Rest day/slide day	Rest day/slide day
T	#39	Off	1:00 hr. Z2 (at 40 min. insert 15 min. Z4)
W	Off	Trans: 30 min. Z2 (QC)	15 min. Z2
R	Off	60 min. Z2 (at 40 min. insert 15 min. Z4)	Off
F	#40	Off	Off
S	Off	3:00 hr. Z2	Off
S	Off	Off	1:30 hr. Z1 to Z2
Totals: 8:45 hr.	1:30 hr.	4:30 hr.	2:45 hr.
WEEK 9	SWIM	BIKE	RUN
M	Rest day/ slide day	Rest day/slide day	Rest day/slide day
T	#41	Off	1:00 hr. Z2 (at 40 min. insert 15 min. Z4)
W	Off	Trans: 30 min. Z2 (QC)	15 min. Z2
R	Off	60 min. Z2 (at 40 min. insert 15 min. Z4)	Off
F	#42	Off	Off
S	Off	3:00 hr. Z2	Off
S	Off	Off	2:00 hr. Z1 to Z2
Totals: 9:15 hr.	1:30 hr.	4:30 hr.	3:15 hr.

WEEK 10	SWIM	BIKE	RUN
M	Rest day/ slide day	Rest day/slide day	Rest day/slide day
T	#43	Off	1:00 hr. Z2 (at 40 min. insert 15 min. Z4)
W	Off	Trans: 45 min. Z2 (QC)	15 min. Z2
R	Off	60 min. Z2 (at 40 min. insert 15 min. Z4)	Off
F	#44	Off	Off
S	Off	3:00 hr. Z2	Off
S	Off	Off	1:45 hr. Z1 to Z2
Totals: 9:15 hr.	1:30 hr.	4:45 hr.	3:00 hr.

Swim Sessions for the Just-Finish Program

Our swims through the first ten weeks will all be approximately 2,000 yards or meters in length, which is a workout distance most athletes can complete within 45 minutes. Our suggestion is that if you need to lengthen the session to last 45 minutes, simply extend the warm-up and/or cooldown portion as needed. If, however, you find you need to shorten the session to make it fit into 45 minutes, reduce the main sets as needed, but keep the warm-up, drills, and cooldown the same.

See page 114 for the numbered swim sessions to be used with this training program.

Peak Training and Taper Phases: Weeks Eleven through Twenty

The second ten weeks (weeks eleven through twenty) of the Just-Finish Program includes both the peak training phase and the taper phase. Our weekly training hours will be at the ten-hour level and we will maintain about 30 to 45 minutes of combined weekly cycling and running Z4 training for most weeks in this phase.

During the second ten weeks we will continue to include two swims of about one hour (2,500 yards/meters) each per week.

Our longest sessions in the second ten weeks will be a five-hour bike session and a three-hour long run.

In the twelfth week we will have a Half Iron-Distance tune-up race. While we should race this event to the best of our ability, our primary purpose is to use this opportunity to practice all of our race-day routines and logistics. This includes pre-race, race, and post-race fueling and hydration; race equipment, and race clothing. We want to test everything out just like we plan to do it for our actual Iron-Distance triathlon. We will identify any elements that we need to adjust prior to the big day and completing this Half Iron-Distance race will provide us with extra confidence and experience as we head into our final eight weeks of preparation.

With three weeks to go before our Iron-Distance race, we will transition into our crisp taper phase to have us rested, sharp, and race-ready. Our durations and higher-intensity training will gradually decrease. Within the final nine days before our race we will not have any training intensities higher than Z2. At this point the hay is in the barn and it is time to taper smart and become physically and mentally energized.

Following is the ten-week peak training and taper phase of the Just-Finish Program:

Adjusting Training Program for Missed Workouts and Other Program Adjustment Tips

See pages 136 and 137 for suggestions on how best to adjust the training programs in this book for missed workouts, plus other great program adjustment tips.

JUST-FINISH PROGRAM — PEAK TRAINING AND TAPER PHASES

WEEK 11	SWIM	BIKE	RUN
M	Rest day/ slide day	Rest day/slide day	Rest day/slide day
T	#45	Off	1:00 hr. Z2 (at 40 min. insert 15 min. Z4)
W	Off	Trans: 30 min. Z2 (QC)	15 min. Z2
R	Off	60 min. Z2 (at 40 min. insert 15 min. Z4)	Off
F	#46	Off	Off
S	Off	3:45 hr. Z2	Off
S	Off	Off	1:30 hr. Z1 to Z2
Totals: 9:30 hr.	1:30 hr.	5:15 hr.	2:45 hr.

WEEK 12	SWIM	BIKE	RUN
M	Rest day/ slide day	Rest day/slide day	Rest day/slide day
T	0.5 hr. easy	Off	45 min. Z1 to Z2 (at 10 min., insert 5 x 1 min. PU @ 1 min. jog)
W	Off	Trans: 45 min. Z1 to Z2 (QC)	15 min. Z1 to Z2
R	Off	60 min. Z1 (at 10 min., insert 5 x 1 min. PU @ 1 min. spin)	Off
F	0.5 hr. easy	Off	Off
S	Off	15 min. Z1—easy bike safety check	30 min. Z1—easy (in a.m.)
S	Race!! Half Iron-Distance	Race!! Half Iron-Distance	Race!! Half Iron-Distance
Totals: 4:30+ hr.	1:00 hr. (+R)	2:00 hr. (+Race)	1:30 hr. (+Race)

JUST-FINISH PROGRAM — PEAK TRAINING AND TAPER PHASES

WEEK 13	SWIM	BIKE	RUN
M	Rest day/slide day	Rest day/slide day	Rest day/slide day
T	#47	Off	60 min. Z1-easy
W	Off	Trans: 30 min. Z2 (QC)	15 min. Z2
R	Off	60 min. Z2	Off
F	#48	Off	Off
S	Off	3:45 hr. Z2	Off
S	Off	Off	2:00 hr. Z1 to Z2
Totals: 10:00 hr.	1:30 hr.	5:15 hr.	3:15 hr.

WEEK 14	SWIM	BIKE	RUN
M	Rest day/slide day	Rest day/slide day	Rest day/slide day
T	#49	Off	1:00 hr. Z2 (at 40 min. insert 15 min. Z4)
W	Off	Trans: 30 min. Z2 (QC)	15 min. Z2
R	Off	60 min. Z2 (at 40 min. insert 15 min. Z4)	Off
F	#50	Off	Off
S	Off	3:15 hr. Z2	Off
S	Off	Off	2:30 hr. Z1 to Z2
Totals: 10:00 hr.	1:30 hr.	4:45 hr.	3:45 hr.

WEEK 15	SWIM	BIKE	RUN
M	Rest day/ slide day	Rest day/slide day	Rest day/slide day
T	#51	Off	1:00 hr. Z2 (at 40 min. insert 15 min. Z4)
W	Off	Trans: 30 min. Z2 (QC)	15 min. Z2
R	Off	60 min. Z2 (at 40 min. insert 15 min. Z4)	Off
F	#52	Off	Off
S	Off	5:00 hr. Z2	Off
S	Off	Off	45 min. Z1 to Z2
Totals: 10:00 hr.	1:30 hr.	6:30 hr.	2:00 hr.
WEEK 16	SWIM	BIKE	RUN
M	Rest day/ slide day	Rest day/slide day	Rest day/slide day
T	#53	Off	1:00 hr. Z2 (at 40 min. insert 15 min. Z4)
W	Off	Trans: 45 min. Z2 (QC)	15 min. Z2
R	Off	60 min. Z2 (at 35 min. insert 20 min. Z4)	Off
F	#54	Off	Off
S	Off	2:30 hr. Z2	Off
S	Off	Off	3:00 hr. Z1 to Z2
Totals: 10:00 hr.	1:30 hr.	4:15 hr.	4:15 hr.

JUST-FINISH PROGRAM — PEAK TRAINING AND TAPER PHASES

WEEK 17	SWIM	BIKE	RUN
M	Rest day/ slide day	Rest day/slide day	Rest day/slide day
T	#55	Off	60 min. Z2 (at 40 min., insert 15 min. Z4)
W	Off	Trans: 45 min. Z2 (QC)	15 min. Z2
R	Off	60 min. Z2 (at 35 min. insert 20 min. Z4)	Off
F	#56	Off	Off
S	Off	5:00 hr. Z2	Off
S	Off	Off	30 min. Z1 to Z2
Totals: 10:00 hr.	1:30 hr.	6:45 hr.	1:45 hr.

WEEK 18	SWIM	BIKE	RUN
M	Rest day/ slide day	Rest day/slide day	Rest day/slide day
T	#57	Off	60 min. Z2 (at 40 min. insert 15 min. Z4)
W	Off	Trans: 45 min. Z2 (QC)	15 min. Z2
R	Off	60 min. Z2 (at 35 min. insert 20 min. Z4)	Off
F	#58	Off	Off
S	Off	3:30 hr. Z2	Off
S	Off	Off	2:00 hr. Z1 to Z2
Totals: 10:00 hr.	1:30 hr.	5:15 hr.	3:15 hr.

WEEK 19	SWIM	BIKE	RUN
M	Rest day/ slide day	Rest day/slide day	Rest day/slide day
T	#59	Off	60 min. Z2 (at 45 min., insert 10 min. Z4)
W	Off	Trans: 45 min. Z2 (QC)	15 min. Z2
R	Off	60 min. Z2 (at 45 min., insert 10 min. Z4)	Off
F	#60	Off	Off
S	Off	2:00 hr. Z2	Off
S	Off	Off	1:00 hr. Z1 to Z2
Totals: 7:30 hr.	1:30 hr.	3:45 hr.	2:15 hr.
WEEK 20	SWIM	BIKE	RUN
M	Rest day/ slide day	Rest day/slide day	Rest day/slide day
T	0.5 hr. easy	Off	45 min. Z1 to Z2 (at 10 min., insert 5 x 1 min. PU @ 1 min. jog)
W	Off	Trans: 30 min. Z1 to Z2 (QC)	15 min. Z1 to Z2
R	Off	45 min. Z1 (at 10 min., insert 5 x 1 min. PU @ 1 min. spin)	Off
F	0.5 hr. easy	Off	Off
S	Off	15 min. Z1—easy bike safety check	30 min. Z1—easy (in a.m.)
S	Race!!	Race!! Iron-Distance	Race!! Iron-Distance
Totals: 4:00+ hr.	1:00 hr. (+R)	1:30 hr. (+Race)	1:30 hr. (+Race)

CHAPTER 13

Transition Strategies for Women

I'm inspired by failure . . .
picking yourself back up again is the
hardest thing in the world.

—*Lolo Jones, track & field, and bobsled athlete*

As experienced triathletes know, triathlons have two transition phases of the race. The first is referred to as "T1" and is when the athlete changes from swimming gear to cycling gear between the swim and bike portions of the race. The second transition is known as "T2," and it is when the athlete changes from cycling gear to running gear. These transitions are some of the most challenging portions of the race. A lot can go wrong during transitions, and the inexperienced triathlete can spoil her entire race due to a host of easy-to-make "rookie mistakes."

Because of the complexity of transitions, they are often referred to as the fourth sport in triathlon. This needs to be fully understood and trained for just like the three main sports. And as is pretty much true with all aspects of triathlon, transitions are no different: Women have their own set of additional transition challenges.

While there are always two transition areas, they can be set up in several different ways, depending on the race. Some races will have the same transition area used for both T1 and T2 and allow the athletes to place their bikes on the bike rack and place gear next to their bikes. This is usually the easiest to prepare for because all of your gear is in one place and you can arrange it however you prefer.

On the other hand, some races have a different area for each transition, and some require you to put your equipment in an equipment bag that is retrieved as you enter the transition area, as opposed to being able to arrange your equipment at the bike rack.

Finally, some races have a combination of the two. For example, you can set up all of your cycling gear with your bike in T1, but then upon entering T2, you have to retrieve your T2 bag with your equipment inside of it.

When you are using equipment bags, there are usually two possibilities. Some races have a changing tent available for you to take your transition bag and change in before retrieving your bike and heading out on the course. This offers the most privacy; however, it is more common to see changing tents with Iron-Distance and other Long Course Races, not the shorter races. Changing tents usually also have access to restrooms, which also provides additional privacy.

The more likely scenario is that you have to take your transition bag with you to the bike rack and change there. This obviously provides less privacy, plus public nudity is not permitted in North America and at many other races around the world.

The type of transitions your race is going to have is not that important. They are all fun challenges. The important thing is that you know well in advance what they are and you make good clothing and equipment choices based on this information. You should practice your transitions in the same format prior to the race.

These challenges include changing race clothing in semi-public "changing tents," the need to use port-a-johns, chafing issues with some types of triathlon clothing, and many more.

Tops-Down/Bottoms-Up Approach

When it comes to efficient transitions, you need a plan. If you do not have a plan, you will be surprised at how difficult it will be to quickly change everything that needs to be changed during the frenzy of transition. We need to have a well-thought-out plan of exactly what we will take off and in what order and what we will put on and in what order. Then, by practicing it and making it second nature, we can do it calmly and efficiently no matter how crazy the transition area is. It's not that important exactly what your plan is, as long as you are comfortable with it and have practiced it frequently enough to do it quickly and correctly.

Many of our coached athletes prefer our "top-down/bottom-up" transition technique. The basic approach is to remove items from your body from top to bottom and then to put them back on in reverse order, from the bottom to the top. This approach provides a nice orderly sequence that is easy to remember.

For example, as you run from the swim finish to T1, remove your goggles, swim cap, and unzip your wet suit. If possible, you can even pull your arms and hands out of the sleeves as you go. When you arrive at your bike in the transition area, remove your wet suit and then begin to put on your cycling gear from the bottom up.

Note that this same approach applies if you are wearing a speed suit instead of a wet suit.

Put your socks on first, if you plan to wear socks. Next put on your cycling shoes (if you are not attaching your shoes to your pedals in advance). We generally suggest most athletes wear a one- or two-piece tri suit for the duration of the race, so no change is required. Next comes your race belt if you are wearing one. Next comes your cycling helmet—buckle it right away (**Tip:** Don't ever forget this one. Besides being extremely important for safety reasons, it's usually an automatic DQ if you forget to buckle!) Finally, put on your sunglasses.

This is a nice efficient and easy-to-remember order. Swimming gear comes off from top to bottom, and cycling gear goes on from bottom to top.

Similarly, as you enter T2 after the bike ride, remove your cycling gear starting from the top and put on your running gear from the bottom up. First, rack your bike (or hand it off to the proper race official) after you safely dismount. Then, as you run toward your bike rack location (or designated changing area), remove your cycling helmet and sunglasses, unless you plan on wearing the same pair of sunglasses on the run. Once you arrive at your bike rack (or designated changing area), remove your cycling shoes and socks, if you are wearing them and unless you plan to wear the same socks for the run. Then put on your running socks and shoes. Next, make sure that your race number is in place. Finally, put on your race cap and sunglasses.

Tip: Notice how the glasses are last. This means that you will not drip on them while attending to your shoes and other lower body items. They will be dry, clear, and good to go.

Just like in T1, this T2 approach is a nice, efficient, and easy-to-remember order. Cycling gear came off from top to bottom, and running gear went on after from bottom to top.

As we said earlier, the tops-down/bottoms-up method is just one possible approach.

How to Train for Transitions

We suggest practicing your transitions with actual race clothing and equipment at least once a week. As little as just 15 minutes will work wonders. This is all "free time."

We like to do what we call "Front-Yard Transitions." Set up your T1 and T2 in your front yard or driveway with your race equipment and clothing just like you plan to on race day. Use race bags if that is what the race will be using. Otherwise, just set up your equipment like you plan to on race day.

Then, put your wet suit on and jog into your T1 setup. Complete T1 as quickly and as efficiently as you can, and then jog back away from the area just like you will on race day. Then, loop back around and come right back to your T2 area. "Rack your bike" as you plan to on race day, and then quickly and efficiently change into your running clothes. Then jog away just as you plan to on race day.

Do this whole sequence completely through twice. Again, the entire session, including setup and breakdown, should take about 15 minutes or less.

Tips: Consider timing yourself each week when you do this to simulate the time pressure of an actual race and also to gauge your improvement over time. Also, consider taking a video of yourself completing your practice transition periodically and view it to see if you can notice areas for improvement.

The Transition Game

Another helpful and fun way to practice your transitions is by playing the transition game. To play, all you need to have is your racing gear and a few of your tri-buddies who also want to improve their transitions.

Establish two or more teams of three to four athletes and set up a transition area with an orange road cone positioned about 50 feet away. The first athlete from each team starts in the transition area dressed in their swim gear and runs to the cone, circles it, and runs back to the transition area. The athlete changes from swim to bike gear and again runs to the cone, circles it, and runs back to the transition area. After the change from bike to running gear, the athlete runs to the cone again, circles it, and runs back to the transition area. Once there, the next member of their team repeats the same sequence. All four team members complete the same sequence in this relay race format. The first team to have all four team members complete the transitions wins.

One of the great benefits of this game is that it provides great transition practice. It simulates the time pressure of an actual race, making it much more real to the athlete.

The second great benefit of the game is that it proves to the athlete the importance of practicing transitions. If the same two teams play several rounds of the game in a row, they almost always become faster with each round. And not just a little faster—they usually become a lot faster. This is simply the result of practice. Each time we repeat steps, we become faster and more efficient at doing them.

If you have an opportunity, get some of your triathlete friends together and play the transition game. Besides improving your transition skills, it's also a blast. You will all have a fun time doing it.

Women-Specific Transition Issues

Following are three special transition issues that are unique to women:

1. Chafing issues

Chafing is a common challenge in endurance racing. The best medicine is a bit of prevention. Start by wearing only wicking fabrics and test them in training. If you are prone to blistering and chafing around your sports bra, armpits, or in your lower half (e.g., labia, perineum, thighs, and butt cheeks) in training it will more than likely occur during a race as well. So, before the race apply a layer of lubrication like Body Glide to all those areas. In transition, depending on the length of the race, you may want or need to reapply lubrication especially in the bike to run transition. There is no shame in applying Body Glide or other lubricant to your privates or other areas so long as you aren't flashing anyone in transition.

2. Bathroom issues

There are a few issues here to discuss. First, if you often need to use the bathroom while you train, you will more than likely need to during a race. So be sure to purchase the proper triathlon racing suit that will make this task as easy as possible. Usually a two-piece tri suit is preferred over a one-piece. Another issue to consider is if you have an incontinence issue or you have your period and need to wear a tampon or pad. You want to be sure your tri suit can accommodate both these situations and you carry an extra pad or tampon with you if necessary. You even want to consider putting a moist wipe in your transition area in case you need to do a little cleanup in the port-a-john. And lastly, always consider the color of your tri suit if this is an issue for you. If you have your period or you often experience leakage or you have to eliminate, white probably isn't the color for you. Go with black—it is a much safer bet. As one of our coached athletes recently said, "I'd love to be able to wear a pink tri suit, but that just may not turn out so well!"

3. **Issues with sports bras and tri suits**

This relates back to both of the above issues. For larger breasted women— and even smaller—a triathlon suit often does not have enough support built in and you will have to wear a sports bra underneath. This can lead to chafing issues so consider the above advice, and also wear the sports bra when you are trying on the suits to make sure the suit is big enough to accommodate it. For some women, a triathlon suit with a built-in bra is all you need. No matter what your choice, please test it out in a longer training session to see how it performs and to see if you experience any chafing.

We hope these tips, guidance, and suggestions help you to maximize your transition performances.

CHAPTER 14

Technique Tips for Female Triathletes

The ladder of success is best climbed by
stepping on the rungs of opportunity.

—Ayn Rand

You might consider the sport of triathlon a double-edged sword. On the
one hand, the beauty of the sport is that there are so many aspects to it
that keep it very interesting, but on the other hand, for that same reason,
it can be overwhelming in knowing how much you need to learn.

To become a successful triathlete, one must learn the basic techniques of
swimming, cycling, and running. Over the years what we have found is that a
lot more triathletes come from a running background rather than swimming
or cycling backgrounds. And as we all know, running is usually something
we have done all of our lives—maybe not in a competitive situation, but
you first learn to crawl, then walk, then run. For swimming and cycling, it's
another story.

So let's break this down into some of the key aspects and techniques of
the three sports and how to go about learning and incorporating good technique in both training and racing.

Swimming Technique from Racing to Training

We'll start with the first sport of the triathlon: swimming. If you are one of
those lucky triathletes who swam in high school or college, you probably
look at triathlon and say, "Great, we start the race with a sport I'm very comfortable with!" For the rest of the athletes, swimming can cause a lot of consternation when done in a mass start or an age-group start with hundreds of
swimmers embarking in the water at the same time.

You are not alone. The majority of athletes look upon the swim start with a level of anxiety much greater than biking and running. And don't let your male counterparts fool you: They experience the same issues. Unless you were an open-water competitive swimmer, this is a totally normal reaction.

A few things you can do to help alleviate the stress of an open-water swim in a triathlon are as follows:

- **Practice swimming in the open water:** Find a triathlete or swim coach to give you a lesson or two in the open water. It will be the best money you will spend. Not only will it help to ease your anxiety, but you will also learn the basics of open-water swimming like learning to sight off the buoys in a race or the shoreline, or learning how to translate your pool swimming to open water.
- **Buy or rent a wet suit to practice with:** Not only is a wet suit helpful in elevating your body in the water, but it is also a flotation device. A wet suit can be 5 millimeters thick, and if you just lie on your back with your belly up, it will keep you above the water. This is hugely comforting to know should you have an anxiety or panic attack.
- **Join an open-water swim group:** Hook up with a triathlon group or club that does weekly swims in a lake or river nearby so you have a group to swim with and you can practice regularly. Most important, never swim alone. You should always have a swim buddy and you should stay within a few feet of each other.
- **Participate in local open-water swim competitions:** Enter a local swim race at the beach or in a lake. You can find open-water swims through your local US Masters Swimming organization (usms.org). Here in New Jersey, we are fortunate to have many opportunities to do a race or two in the spring or summertime, usually about 1 or 2 miles in length, which is great practice for any triathlon distance.

Pool Swimming Technique

Again, if you were a swimmer in high school or college, or just a good swimmer, your best bet is to join a local Masters Swim team and swim a few times with them. It's a great way to push yourself and swim a little more than you would on your own. Also, it is a great way to practice swimming with a group of swimmers similar to a race situation.

The other benefit of swimming on a Masters Swim team is you can usually ask the coach for pointers and advice on your stroke. This will help you to focus on your weaknesses and continue to improve over time.

If you are not comfortable swimming in a class, then you might want to consider going to a local swim coach to take some one-on-one swim lessons first.

So, what are the basics of swimming and what should you focus on? One of the big differences we find between men and women in swimming is their ability to balance in the water. Generally, women are more relaxed and have an easier time finding their balance in the water, but let's expand on that further.

Balance

We like to use the analogy of a seesaw when swimming. If you think of your chest as the middle of the seesaw, and your hands and feet as the ends of the seesaw, it may help you to understand balance in the water. If you push flat on your chest off the wall in a pool, there should be slight pressure on your sternum while pointing your arms downward in the water and keeping your head aligned with your spine. By doing this, your lower body should become elevated and level on the water. When your body is level on the water, it creates the least amount of drag through the water, which is very important because water is much denser than air.

Head Position and Breathing

We highlight your head position because it is very important that your head be aligned with your spine, just like good posture, in order to properly maintain good balance and efficient breathing.

If you were to push off the wall and raise your head to see where you are going, you will cause drag in the water by creating a larger surface area. If you push your head too far down in the water and submerge it, you will likely create more drag because you will have to lift your head to breathe, thus causing your feet to sink. What you do with your head will often dictate what is happening with your legs and feet.

First and foremost, you should begin a slow exhalation as soon as your mouth touches the water and continue your exhalation until you turn your head to breathe. When breathing, you want to be sure to keep your ear in the water, along with one goggle, as you turn your head. You want to pull your eyes down like you are looking under your armpit and slightly behind you, without lifting your head out of the water.

Body Position and Rotation

So beyond the position of our head, we must also be aware of our body position in the freestyle stroke. In freestyle, you are constantly trying to get to the narrowest position you can in the water. We often use the analogy of being on a skewer. Your head remains steady and your shoulders and hips rotate side to side. Your hips rotate further than your shoulders. You want to make sure when you rotate your shoulders you do not go beyond your armpit. Envision swimming from armpit, across your chest, to your other armpit. However, once you get to that position in the front, your hips continue to rotate slightly farther.

A good land technique to try is to stand in front of a wall with your nose touching the wall. Then take your left hand and with your fingers, crawl up the wall straight from your shoulder until your armpit is flat to the wall. Simultaneously, using your obliques and abs, rotate your hips to the right and take your right front foot and bring it behind your left foot, keeping your leg just slightly bent. Repeat this movement several times on one side and then the other. This is your narrowest profile and a position you want to try to obtain in the water. In freestyle, you should be going from side to side in that position as smoothly as possible. For most women, we are much wider at our hips than our shoulders so it's even more important we learn to maximize our rotation in our lower half.

Recovery

Now that we know how our head and body should be positioned in the water to achieve an efficient freestyle stroke, what is the best technique for recovery? The recovery begins when your hand exits the water at or near your thigh and lasts until your hand reenters the water beyond your head.

Since there is nothing to be gained in the recovery, you want to use your shoulder to raise your arm up from your body with your elbow bent and your hand relaxed under it to just beyond your head. A good cue is to lead the recovery with your elbow until your hand gets beyond your head, and then you can extend your hand and arm into the water.

From our experience, this seems to be more difficult for women compared to men. The reason we have found is that most women are not as strong in their upper back and arms and often drop their elbows and try to recover with their hands. Always remember, your elbow should be higher than your hand in all aspects of the stroke.

Catch and Pull

After your hand enters the water, you should extend it almost straight while keeping your armpit and palm flat to the floor of the pool (i.e., do not overextend your arm so you turn onto your back, or turn your hand so your thumb is pointed toward the ceiling).

You begin the catch with the extended arm by bending at your elbow and bringing your hand perpendicular to the floor of the pool, and your palm facing back, thus creating a paddle from the middle of your bicep to your fingertips. This movement is to catch the water. As your hips simultaneously rotate further, you are pulling your hand through the water underneath your body and toward your belly button. Once underneath your belly button, you finish the stroke by pushing the water so your hand finishes close to your thigh as though you were flexing your triceps.

These are the basic components of freestyle and elements you should try to master. To help you do that, here are three drills that we find are most helpful in mastering the freestyle stroke:

Kick on Side Progression Drill

We recommend you use swim fins to perform this drill most efficiently and effectively. This is a great drill that will help you with body position, relaxed recovery, good body rotation, and focus on the catch and pull.

1. **First progression:** Begin with one arm extended in front of you with your armpit and palm flat in the water and your arm tilted downward about 6 to 10 inches under the water, while your other arm remains on your side with your hand closer to the front of your thigh. Your head should be in alignment with your spin and can be slightly submerged for purposes of this drill. Push off the wall flat on your stomach, then rotate your hips toward the wall, head facing down, and kick across the pool. When you need to

breathe, take a breath by turning your head until your mouth clears the water before returning your head to its facedown position. Repeat that with your other arm extended on the return length.

2. **Second progression—stroke with one arm:** Perform the same drill above; simultaneously, while taking a breath, begin the recovery part of the stroke with the arm that is at your side. Take a full stroke, only stopping again when your arm returns to your thigh. On the return length, repeat with the opposite arm extended and stroke with the other arm.

3. **Third progression—alternate two strokes each side:** Perform the same drill above except after stroking twice with one arm, rotate all the way to the other side and take two strokes with the other arm. For this progression, take a breath only on the first stroke on each side. Try not to take a breath on both strokes on both sides. Be sure to fully rotate between each stroke, and keep the lead arm in front in the palm-down position until the recovering arm has reached it.

4. **Fourth Progression—almost swimming or delayed swimming:** Perform this drill the same as the third progression except only take one stroke before switching to the other side and taking a stroke with the other arm. It's really important that the lead arm remain in front until the recovering arm has reached it out in front.

One Arm Progression Drill with One Arm at Your Side

This drill focuses on so many important elements, from working on proper breathing to fluid body rotation to efficient catch and pull. It allows you to work on each of these elements, isolated one at a time.

1. **First progression:** Start with one arm at your side and the other out in front. You are going to swim as though you only have one arm. Push off the wall and rotate your hips opposite the arm that is extended. If your left arm is extended, rotate your hips to the right and begin kicking. Take a breath to the right (opposite your extended arm), bring your head back facedown into the water as you begin to rotate your hips and torso to the opposite side. Once your hips are fully rotated to the opposite side, take a full stroke

with the extended arm. As your hand reenters the water, begin to rotate your hips back to the opposite side of your extended arm to the start position. Repeat this position by taking a breath first. On the return length, switch arms.

2. **Second progression:** Perform this drill the same way as the first progression, except add "fingertip drag" during the recovery portion of the stroke. Fingertip drag is when you raise your elbow straight up along your body line with your hand relaxed under your elbow, while keeping your fingertips in contact with the water as you recover.

3. **Third progression:** Same as the first progression, except perform two strokes with one arm and then switch and perform two strokes with the other arm, while smoothing transitioning from side to side. Be sure to keep the opposite arm at your side for the two strokes and then recover with the opposite arm as you rotate toward that side, and then perform two strokes with that arm. This can be a tricky drill, but keep practicing as it is a great way to get smooth in the water, learn your balance, and find your power.

Pull Buoy Progression Drill

We are not much for "pool toys," but what we have found is that some gadgets in the water can be helpful. The pull buoy, which is a device that you normally place between your thighs at crotch height, is used to help you elevate your legs in the water and also helps with rotation and building some upper body swim-specific strength. As we mentioned earlier, a lot of women have a weaker upper body and less developed swim-specific muscles than men. This drill progression is helpful in developing some strength but also helpful in learning good rotation in the water (i.e., learning to get our hips out of the way). We will perform this drill without fins.

1. **First progression:** You want to put your goggles on before placing the pull buoy between your ankles. Then push off the wall flat on your stomach with both hands in front and begin taking a stroke with one arm. You must first rotate your hips to the side that you are stroking without losing your balance on your opposite armpit

or else the pull buoy will take over and you will end up on your back. It may take a couple of tries but give it a chance. You must keep your nonstroking arm in front and pointed downward in the water, while you rotate your opposite hips to the side so you can take a stroke and then begin alternating strokes with each arm.

The pull buoy forces an even rotation of your hips side to side and helps you to hold your balance in the water while you are breathing and stroking. We recommend you take a few strokes before you take your first breath so you get a good rhythm of rotation through your hips from side to side.

2. **Second progression:** The same drill as above, except move the pull buoy to just below your knees and repeat the drill above.

3. **Third progression:** The same drill as above, except move the pull buoy to crotch height and perform the same drill.

This series of drills with the pull buoy will help you to gain not only physical strength but also help you learn to be fluid in the water and avoid over-rotation, especially while breathing.

Once you have mastered the swim drills that use fins, try them without the fins!

Cycling Technique

While swimming is very technique oriented, cycling is not to the same extent. Cycling has been around for more than a century, and aside from the technological advances in gearing and shifting, the bike still has to be powered by you.

Once you have familiarized yourself with the basic components of the bike, it is time to get on it and ride. As with swimming, it is all about holding good posture on the bike to pedal with the maximum efficiency and power.

Some of the common issues we see with women reside in their bike-handling skills, especially their climbing and descending skills. The former is usually due to fear of getting out of the saddle and the latter is fear of falling on a downhill. These are all valid feelings, but these fears can be overcome with good technique and practice.

Posture

Let's start with good posture on the bike. Once you get on your bike, start by sitting straight up on your bike with a flat back. Then sort of fall forward and place your hands over your brake hoods while keeping your elbows slightly bent. You want to avoid locking out your elbows and white knuckling your hands on the handlebars.

You want to keep your back flat at 45°. As you may have experienced, as your extend your time on the bike in a session, your form starts to deteriorate. You may find that when you're tired, you allow yourself to relax your core and your back rounds. Or you tighten your grip on the handlebars and lock out your elbows, thus causing stress to your neck and shoulders. So, it is important you focus on your form all the while you are riding.

Cadence

What we have found with a lot of women is they will push either too hard of a gear or too easy of a gear, for one reason or another. You want to learn to spin your pedals in a circle as opposed to mashing your pedals by pushing down too hard and then toeing down too much to pull up on the pedals. A good visualization for learning to spin is to imagine you are scraping dog poop off the bottom of your shoe from the 4 o'clock to the 7 o'clock position. Below is a great diagram of how your foot should be positioned as you pedal a circle.

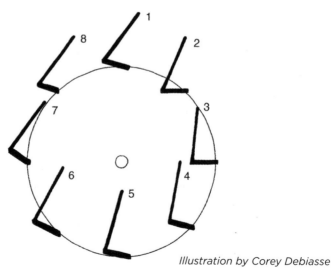

Illustration by Corey Debiasse

In general, you want to keep your cadence between 75 and 105 revolutions per minute (rpm), depending on the terrain. When climbing, it's normal for your cadence to drop to under 80 rpm, but you want to try to maintain a higher cadence for as long as possible. While descending, you may not be pedaling at all, or at a higher cadence of over 100 rpm. And on a long stretch of flat road, most women can maintain a cadence of 90 to 95 with a moderate Z2 heart rate, and at about 80 rpm when maintaining a higher-intensity Z4 heart rate. There are many different opinions as to the ideal cadence, but this is what we have found works well for most women.

Climbing Technique

This is an area that a lot of women find the most difficult to learn but once they do, they can become great climbers! And if there is one thing a guy hates, it is to be "chicked" climbing a hill. So if you want to have some fun with your male training buddies, learn to climb—it can be so much fun.

Since most women are more comfortable sitting in the saddle than getting out of the saddle, women are better seated climbers as women draw most of their strength from their glutes and legs. But this isn't to say that women should not learn how to climb a hill out of the saddle.

When you approach a hill, you want to shift into a lower (easier) gear, possibly even less of a gear than you think you need. You do not want to get stuck having to shift once on the hill as you risk dropping your chain. As you reach the midpoint of the climb, your cadence will continue to drop but your goal is to try to maintain your speed and cadence for as long as you can.

Since most women find the seated position easier to master, force yourself to stand more often than you prefer on a hill so you can practice that technique as well.

To stand during a hill climb, you must first shift up one or two gears (harder) and then stand. You want to straighten your arms slightly to rock the bike in a straight line side to side underneath you by pulling up on one side and pushing down with your pedal on the other side. A lot of women try to use their arms to power the bike, which is not what you want to do. Your pelvis should be forward so you are not standing straight up on your pedals. You should be in a position that feels like your knees are going to hit your handlebars. Keep your wrists flexible and avoid gripping the handlebars too tightly. Use your legs to power the bike.

Generally, for a hill that takes 1 minute or less to climb, you should be able to stay seated and power over the hill. For a climb that takes about 1 to 4 minutes, you will want to try to remain seated for about two-thirds of it and then stand for the last third of the climb. And for climbs that will take more than 4 minutes, alternate between sitting and standing to help keep your leg muscles fresher.

This is definitely a skill that takes time to learn, so be diligent and practice it with every ride you do. The more you practice it, the easier it will come.

Descending

For a lot of women, descending can be tougher than climbing. The fear factor of being able to stop quickly or losing control of your bike is real. And compared to your male counterparts, it is good to have a certain level of fear when descending to avoid carelessness that can ultimately result in a crash.

However, if you are going to ride in a triathlon, you have to learn how to descend comfortably and safely. We recommend you start by practicing on a small hill on a quiet street with little to no traffic.

You want to put your weight flat on the seat, centered over the rear tire. If you have aero bars or are using your drops, and you are fully comfortable with them, now is the time to put them to use. If you aren't, then keep your hands on the brake hoods so you can feather them to slow down to a speed you are comfortable with on the descent.

You want to keep your pedals at the 3 and 9 o'clock positions to be more aerodynamic as you descend and to avoid anything coming up from the road and hitting your pedals. If you are comfortable descending, this is a great way to gain time on your competitors.

If you are afraid of descending, try to befriend the enemy by practicing often and every time you ride. The more comfortable you become on your bike, the more comfortable you will be in race conditions.

Cornering

In our experience, most triathletes—women especially—sit up going around a turn instead of learning proper technique. Cornering is an easy skill to learn, so try to master it. As you approach a turn or corner, you want to try to maintain speed if the severity of the turn allows you to. To do this, you want to straighten the outer leg so it's at the bottom of the pedal stroke (6 o'clock position) and the inner leg is bent, with your knee at a 90-degree angle. Avoid steering the bike into the turn with your hands, but rather use your body weight and knee to lean into the turn. If possible, you want to "cut the apex" of the turn, or ideal line, to keep the shortest distance around it. You have to be careful when doing that to avoid traffic and other riders in a race.

Braking

This is a very important skill to learn, obviously, but one that is often assumed. You need to be ready to come to a complete stop quickly should the situation arise, to avoid a car or pedestrian or anything else. You can practice this while training outside anytime. You want to start by pushing your weight back on the seat and grabbing both brakes at the same time. It's important to know the front brake alone provides the fastest stopping power; however, you have to learn how to apply the front brake hard without having the rear wheel lift off the ground and over your head. You do this by keeping both arms stiff and using them to decelerate while getting your center of gravity far back by pushing back on the saddle.

Cycling Correction and Technique Drills

Single-Leg Pedaling

This is a great drill to practice in the first 15 minutes of a ride as you warm up. It will help you to activate the proper cycling muscles and get you focused on smooth cycling and focused cadence.

Using only one foot, spin the one pedal for 15 to 30 seconds and then switch and spin with the other foot for 15 to 30 seconds. If you are riding outside, you can keep your foot clipped into your pedal but avoid applying any pressure to the foot you are not using. You can do this for several minutes. You will notice almost immediately which leg is stronger and which leg feels more comfortable throughout the spin cycle. It will help you to better learn to spin with the weaker leg and even out your pedaling stroke on both sides.

High-Cadence Cycling

A great way to learn to be efficient in your pedaling is to spin at a high cadence for a period of time like 30 to 60 minutes. This will help you find your balance on the bike and help you find an efficient pedaling stroke.

You can do this drill by spinning at a designated cadence like 100 rpm for a specified period of time. Or you can try spinning at varying cadences at varying intervals of time. For example:

EXAMPLE 1

Repeat one or more times
100 rpm @ 15 min.
105 rpm @ 10 min.
110+ rpm @ 5 min.

EXAMPLE 2

Repeat five or more times
100 rpm @ 3 min.
105 rpm @ 2 min.
110 rpm @ 1 min.

You can try these drills in any of your recovery spins that you find in the training programs in Chapters 10, 11, 12, and 16.

Running Technique

Although most of us learned to run when we were kids, a lot of women have issues running resulting mostly from the natural angles of women. Women tend to have wider hips and this causes what is referred to as the "Q-angle," or the ratio of your hips to your knees. It can result in IT band issues as well as hip, knee, and feet issues.

So, although running is natural for most women, proper technique must be learned. As with swimming and cycling, running is about maintaining good posture. If you lean too far forward or too far back, it can cause a whole host of issues.

Two Strings Concept

A visualization we like to use with our athletes is running like a marionette and our "two-strings" concept. You want to begin in a standing position with your arms relaxed at your sides looking straight ahead. Envision a string coming out of the top of your head pulling you straight up, let your shoulders hang relaxed, and envision another string coming out of your chest, pulling you slightly forward. You can practice this technique in a standing position with your elbows bent and forearms parallel to the ground while your thumbs are softly placed on a closed hand. Then, go up and down onto your toes with the two-strings visualization as you swing your arms back and forth.

Bounceless Running

Oftentimes we see runners who are wasting a lot of energy by going up and down in their running form instead of touching the ground and going forward. If you run like this, you know it, because everything in front of you is bouncing up and down.

A good technique to remediate this problem in conjunction with the two-strings approach is to engage your lower abs by pulling in your belly to achieve a neutral pelvic position. Then begin to take your first strides while holding that position. You will find much less bouncing and more forward momentum, as your hips remain level. This is a good drill to practice on a treadmill in front of a mirror, focusing on keeping your hips level and moving from your legs down.

Running Drills

There are some great running drills to help you improve your running technique as well as ready your body to run. Here are a few that you may want to consider experimenting with as you look to improve your running technique. A good place to do these is on a track, but any flat, safe running surface will do.

Legs Swing Front to Back and Side to Side

This is a great warm-up drill before beginning your run. Start in a standing position with a wall or chair to your side to hold on to. Raise your knee straight up toward your chest and then swing it back as you straighten the leg using your hips to do the swinging like a pendulum. Repeat ten times before switching to the other leg.

Then face forward with enough space between you and the wall or chair to swing your leg out to the side, then let it fall in front of your other leg, across your body. Repeat this ten times, and then switch and do it with the other leg.

Lateral Crossovers

Start with your hips and shoulders facing forward, then take the left leg and cross it behind your right leg, and then bring it in front of your right leg, and repeat for 15 to 30 seconds. Repeat this drill with the right leg leading the exercise.

Heel to Toe to Hop to Run

With your hands clasped behind your head, start by placing one foot in front of the other, striking with your heel and rolling onto your toe, alternating your feet for about ten steps. For the next ten steps, add a hop once you get to your toe. Try to keep your hips level and maintain good posture. For the last part of this drill, drop your arms to your sides in a bent position and run for ten steps while maintaining level hips.

We have given you a lot of tools to help you improve your technique in all three disciplines. Now put these to use and set some goals to improve in the off-season and most important, follow through.

As we began this chapter, we'll end it by saying the beauty of triathlon is the many facets of the sport that keep us motivated, interested, and constantly learning. It is a great sport to challenge both your physical and mental capacities, and even your patience at times.

CHAPTER 15

Health Strategies and Injury Prevention

An ounce of prevention
is worth a pound of cure.

*—Benjamin Franklin, one of the
United States' Founding Fathers*

There are so many aspects to training for a triathlon, and to add to the list are the very common health issues and injuries athletes face in their triathlon journeys. All athletes, whether male or female, have health issues to consider, in addition to remaining injury-free in their quest. However, women typically have a list of potential injuries and health issues that are unique to women and most men will never experience.

We want to learn to face our health issues head on, from getting regular physicals and gynecological exams to recognizing when an injury is coming on and addressing the cause and ultimate remedy.

If you have been in the sport of triathlon for any time, you know you are either one of those triathletes who has been injured or one of those that will be injured at some point. It is pretty much a given, but the fact of the matter is that you can minimize these occurrences with a little bit of effort and focus.

While women experience many of the same injuries in training and racing as men, from ITB syndrome to plantar fasciitis, women have specific health issues to contend with as well. These may include monthly menstrual or menopausal issues like unwanted weight gain. Not to mention the pregnant woman who wants to continue to train and race for as long as possible while pregnant.

Following is a discussion of five of the most common special health issues women face and our suggestions on how best to address them.

1. **Menstrual cycle**

We are sure many of you have woken up the day before your race or on race morning to find out you have your period. It is not exactly what you planned, but you have trained for many months and you are not going to allow this to stop you.

Menstrual cycles affect just about every premenopausal woman and can be a disruption to training and racing. Following are some of the issues you may face or should be aware of and then some suggested remedies:

- **Knee injuries:** Female athletes are between two and eight times more likely to injure their ACL knee ligaments than men. This is due to their monthly menstrual cycle, and while it has been thought to be more prevalent during ovulation, it can be an issue for some women anytime during the cycle.[1]
- **Excessive bleeding:** Excessive bleeding can cause anemia and affect your training and racing performance in that the lack of iron in the blood does not allow for good oxygen transfer to the muscles.
- **Exercise-induced amenorrhea:** This is the absence of monthly periods due primarily to intense exercise. It can cause issues with bone density, irregular periods, lower than normal body weight, and occasional stress fractures.
- **Bloating, cramping, swelling, moodiness:** Most women experience at least one or more of these symptoms either before or during their period due to hormonal changes around your period. It can range from mild to severe and can definitely impact your training and racing.

There are many remedies out there to curb menstrual symptoms and some work for some women and not for others. If you haven't been able to control these symptoms or find any relief from them, here are a few suggestions:

- Be more cautious around your period to avoid any potential ACL issues. Listen to your body, understand your cycle, and use a low-

---

1   Online article: *Menstrual Cycle Affects Knee*, published April 20, 2009, News-Medical.net.

impact cross-training option around your menstruation to avoid a potential knee injury.

- Many women will take extra vitamins and minerals such as calcium, magnesium, vitamin B6, vitamins D and E, and an iron supplement around their monthly period to help combat some of the symptoms of moodiness, cramping, and swelling.
- More often used are NSAIDs to control cramping and headaches so you can get through your training and racing. Be cautious taking them on race day as they can cause potential stomach issues, and always take them with food.
- Other pharmacologic treatments some women use are evening primrose, St. John's wart, and chaste-tree berry to reduce the effects of menstrual cramps, swelling, and moodiness.
- Birth control pills can also be used to manage the timing of menstruation and reduce monthly symptoms like excessive bleeding.

These are just some of the strategies for dealing with your menstrual cycle but you should always check with your gynecologist or doctor first. You should make sure to track your period monthly beginning with ovulation and get a better understanding of how you are affected by it, from your moods to your energy levels. You want to understand your cycle and learn to train around it.

2. **Birth control**

For most women, being on birth control is a nonissue and can actually help you plan your racing schedule to avoid having your period on race day. If you are using any type of birth control, from the pill to an IUD, you can experience negative and positive effects on your training. Following are some of the most common potential negative effects:

- **Blood clotting:** Being on birth control as an athlete, you are potentially at risk of getting a blood clot, mostly due to sitting for long periods; for example, when you fly and you allow yourself to get dehydrated. For endurance athletes, if we are not diligent about it, we can be walking around in a constant dehydrated state. For athletes that travel via airplane for races or for work, this is something you should be very aware of and know the symptoms as well.

- **Sun overexposure:** Some birth control methods can make your skin more sensitive to sunburn and other negative effects of the sun.
- **Fluid retention:** Fluid retention caused by birth control can cause undue bloating and discomfort.

Most of these potential issues can be dealt with pretty easily. Here are some suggestions:

- The same remedies are used by women who are on birth control pills and those who are not, from additional vitamins and NSAIDs and other pharmacological remedies (see above), as those addressing normal menstrual issues.
- Always be sure to wear sunblock when taking birth control pills and avoid prolonged exposure to the sun without appropriate cover. The new sun protection clothing technology is a great way to enjoy training outdoors while avoiding overexposure to the sun.
- Be very careful when flying immediately after a hard workout or race. You may already be experiencing inflammation and swelling and a pressurized cabin will make that worse. A blood clot is a potential if you are dehydrated or you do not get up often enough and move around to keep your blood circulating. You should drink lots of water during travel and avoid drinking alcoholic beverages. Often athletes will wear compression socks while traveling to help maintain good blood circulation.

These are all good remedies, but of course you should check with your gynecologist or doctor to see if these treatments would be helpful and safe for you while you are taking or using any birth control methods.

3. **Pregnancy**

Many of the myths about training during pregnancy have pretty much been debunked, from higher-intensity interval training to keeping your heart rate below 140 beats per minute. Generally, if you are healthy and have been exercising regularly prior to pregnancy, your doctor will more than likely give you the thumbs up to continue doing so. However, there are some things you need to know and be aware of:

- **Increased oxygen consumption:** During pregnancy, as your baby grows, it will require more oxygen and thus you will fatigue sooner than normal.
- **Dehydration:** Pregnant women should increase their normal water intake by about 2 to 3 quarts a day without consideration for exercise, but even more so while exercising. Dehydration risk is much greater for pregnant women when exercising.
- **Caloric intake:** A pregnant woman should consume an additional 300 calories a day just to support the baby normally, without consideration for exercise. If you are continuing to train through pregnancy, you may need to increase your calorie intake even further to avoid losing weight.
- **Dizziness and fatigue:** Dizziness and fatigue can happen more easily when you are pregnant, especially in that first trimester when your body is adjusting to the pregnancy.
- **Balance:** The added weight and distribution of the weight associated with pregnancy can be challenging, especially during exercise.

We all know many women who have continued to train through pregnancy and even race in the early stages without any ill effect. However, always discuss your plans with your doctor and get his or her advice beforehand. These are just a few suggestions and ideas on how to train through pregnancy:

- The general rule of thumb for pregnant women is that if you were a regular exerciser before you got pregnant, you can continue doing that exercise through pregnancy.
- You can do some higher-intensity training, but you want to avoid raising your body temperature too high as you can affect your health and the health of the baby if you get overheated. Exercise indoors, where you can control the temperature, and dress appropriately to help your body regulate your core body temperature.
- Scale back the intensity of your workouts and consult with your doctor as to what you can do throughout the pregnancy. Usually on

a perceived exertion scale (with 1 being the lowest and 10 being the highest), it is recommended that you stay in that 7–8 range. You really need to listen to your body and train how you feel. If you are fatigued or tired one day, back off your training or do something less strenuous like swimming or cycling as opposed to running.

- Use a stationary bike instead of training outdoors on the bike to reduce the risk of a fall or accident, and avoid off-road running where there is potential to trip and fall. Stick with flat, predictable surfaces.
- If you plan to race while pregnant, obviously get your doctor's approval, keep your effort at 70 percent of your normal race effort, and proceed with extreme caution. A fall or accident is not something you want to undergo while pregnant.
- Embrace swimming as it is one of those exercises you can do right up until birthing, and for most women it is the best exercise to compensate for loss of balance as you get further into the pregnancy.

Talk to other athletes who have been in a similar situation to understand potentially what you can expect to do as you progress in the pregnancy. Our experience with women athletes we have trained who were pregnant was that they are usually able to continue training, but at a lower intensity level, and if they continue to race, it is not at the same level. Once into the third trimester, most women find they cannot continue to race, however, they do continue to train at a reduced intensity and duration right up until the baby is born. The benefits of exercising while pregnant are being shown more and more so consult your doctor and listen to your body.

4. **Menopause**

This is a topic we could write pages and pages about simply gathering all the data from our many coached athletes over the years. The average age of women affected by menopause is fifty-one years old, but you can experience symptoms in your forties and symptoms can least for several years or more. There are those women who are greatly affected by menopause and those who skate through it. However, we have found more women having issues than not and they run the gamut. Following are some of the most common symptoms of menopause.

- **Lack of sleep:** Many women who are going through menopause will experience irregular sleep patterns, which will adversely affect their ability and desire to work out. If you are exhausted from lack of sleep, the last thing you want to do is get up and work out.
- **Hot flashes/night sweats:** Hot flashes and night sweats associated with menopause can cause dehydration and loss of electrolytes as well as a decrease in a woman's heat tolerance. The exact cause of hot flashes is not known, but they can be exacerbated by some foods like caffeine and alcohol.
- **Weight gain:** Unwanted weight gain is common as you experience reduced estrogen levels. Additionally, lack of sleep can cause weight gain. As we all know, an additional 5 to 10 pounds can have a negative impact on your training and racing.
- **Bone density:** As your estrogen levels drop, many women will experience bone loss through menopause and well after. This is of great concern for women and something to be addressed with your doctor.
- **Loss of muscle mass:** Another effect of hormonal changes experienced through menopause is a significant loss of muscle mass. This can also be attributed to excess weight gain and potentially give rise to more injuries.
- **Dehydration:** As a woman goes through menopause, there is a resulting thinning of their skin. As a result, dehydration is increased in menopausal women.

These are the things your mother never told you about when you were growing up and things you do not think about until it happens to you. The end result of not having your monthly cycle can be positive. However, getting through that period of change can be a rough road.

Here are some remedies that you may want to experiment with as you go through your menopause battle:

- To reduce the effects of hot flashes, many women have had success with the herb black cohosh. But while it works for some women, it does not work for all.
- Estrogen therapies have proven effective but some can be risky, so you need to work with your doctor to determine which, if any, would

be effective for you. Some of our athletes have used a hormone patch without side effects and it has helped them get through those hormonal imbalances, while continuing to train and race in triathlons.

- As important as it is to stay hydrated, it is even more important for menopausal women. With the thinning of your skin, hot flashes, and night sweats, you can run the risk of getting dehydrated more often than normal. Drink lots of fluids before, during, and after exercise to avoid dehydration.

- Calcium, vitamin D, and dietary calcium from yogurt, cheese, and milk and leafy greens like kale, spinach, and broccoli are all good ways to ensure you have good bone density. While running helps to maintain good bone density, strength training is very important too to maintain bone density, as well as muscle mass. However, consult your doctor and take supplements if necessary because as you age it becomes more difficult for women to absorb those vitamins and nutrients through food.

As with all health issues, discuss them with your doctor or health-care provider so you understand any potential side effects and other issues that could possibly affect your ability to train and race in triathlon.

5. **Self-image and low self-esteem**

Your self-esteem affects how you feel about yourself and how you perceive the world sees you. For many women, although they may never be 100 percent satisfied with their bodies, they do appreciate their genetics and body type and are generally satisfied with their appearance. However, for some women, this is an ongoing battle. It can stem from longtime obesity or low self-esteem as a child and may unfortunately preclude them from even venturing out to try the sport of triathlon. Not only are the physical aspects of triathlon training daunting to some, but so are some of the basic issues associated with triathlon, from the clothing to the outward physical appearance. Some of those issues include the following:

- **Tri suit or swimsuit:** Triathlon clothing can be quite skimpy and is often a deterrent to getting into the sport due to the lack of knowledge of what is available in triathlon clothing for women.

- **Larger women:** Both large breasted women and overweight woman often feel self-conscious and uncomfortable running and biking in general let alone triathlon clothing.
- **Racing with the male gender:** Racing with men can be intimidating and also add to the stress about your appearance.

We have worked with many female athletes, from extremely fit and competitive women to women who have never been inclined to participate in a sport until now. And we can tell you there is great satisfaction in helping all of these women find the courage to do a triathlon.

Here are some points you may not know about triathlon or factors you might not have considered that may help you find your way to the starting line:

- Get yourself to a local triathlon and you will be amazed to see the shapes and sizes of not only the women but also the men that participate in this sport. It's not all the perfect "10" bodies or athletic types you might expect.
- The sport of triathlon is a participation sport and as a result manufacturers have realized the need of athletes of all shapes and sizes from athletic equipment to clothing and shoes. No matter your size or shape, you will be able to find the right triathlon equipment and gear that will work for you and give you the confidence to join the world of triathlon.
- If intimated by men, try a women-only race. It is a great way to meet women triathletes like yourself and avoid the stress of facing men in your first triathlon. You'll find more newbies at these races that you can bond with, and who knows, you may find yourself boosting someone else who needs some encouragement.
- Join a Tri Club that has a supportive group of women that you can travel with to races and who give you that support of knowing someone who is experienced is right there to help you should you need it.
- If the above suggestions still don't work for you, seek professional help to finds ways to address these issues. There are many athletes that use psychologists and psychiatrists to help them deal with the mental aspects of triathlon training and racing.

The bottom line is that the sport of triathlon has been a women's sport from the beginning. It has treated women the same as men but has also embraced the specific needs of women. As with all health issues, always seek the advice of your doctor or health-care provider before attempting any remedies for your symptoms, and talk to other triathletes and friends who have had similar experiences. There is a lot to be gained from others' experiences and avoiding having to reinvent the wheel.

Dealing with Injuries

Most of us have experienced being injured, from a broken bone to a simple overuse injury, and it is not fun! Injuries can result from a lack of proper training or stem from another health issue like menstruation or menopause. The key to dealing with injuries is first to try to prevent them, and second, if they do occur, to address them head on. Get yourself to a qualified doctor and get a diagnosis so you can start to treat the injury immediately.

From our experience coaching many women over the years, probably the most common injuries and potential remedies we see are the following:

1. **Stress fractures:** Stress fractures can be caused by overtraining, low bone density, menopause, menstruation, or improper form or technique. Here are some remedies you might want to consider:
   - You should first see a doctor to confirm the fracture and in most situations you will most likely have to stay off of a lower-extremity stress fracture and avoid any weight-bearing activities.
   - After the initial healing, start back with nonimpact or weight-bearing exercise. Most doctors will recommend swimming and cycling as an entry back into exercise.
   - Find a good physical therapist or Active Release Technique provider in your area who is experienced in treating triathletes and understands your training regimen to help get you back out there training again. And most important, follow through with their recommended stretching and exercise protocol.
   - When you are ready to get back to training, remember, a gradual return to exercise is best and avoiding "too much too soon" is highly recommended. A good coach can design a solid plan so

you can return to your normal level of exercise without getting reinjured.

2. **Iliotibial band syndrome (ITB):** ITB syndrome is a condition that can be caused by overtraining or too much increase in volume, duration, or intensity and improper technique. The primary symptom of ITB syndrome is when you feel pain on the outside of your knee (not the front of your knee). Some of the most basic remedies for ITB syndrome are as follows:
   - RICE = Rest, Ice, Compression, and Elevation to reduce the immediate pain, but continue with icing daily and use anti-inflammatories to reduce the inflammation.
   - Stretching and strengthening your hip area may help as well.
   - Incorporating cross training into your training regimen may help to get you back to regular training but also prevent it from happening to begin with.
   - Seek the advice of a qualified physical therapist or ART (Active Release Technique) provider or orthopedic doctor if you are unsure of the injury and how to deal with it.

3. **Plantar fasciitis:** Plantar fasciitis is one of the most challenging of the injuries because it is so difficult to stay off your feet even if you are not exercising. Therefore, the time it takes to heal can be greatly increased and can remain up to six months. It can be caused by too much exercise too soon or poor running mechanics or just tightness in your calves. Here are some remedies you might want to consider:
   - RICE = Rest, Ice, Compression, and Elevation to reduce the immediate pain from plantar fasciitis, but continue with icing daily and use anti-inflammatories to reduce the inflammation.
   - Stretch your calves three to five times a day with calf-stretching exercises, from dropping your heel off a step or curb to wall stretching with a straight leg.
   - Tape the arch of your foot during exercise and while walking around. Avoid wearing high-heeled shoes or flip-flops as they give little support to the plantar fascia.

- Use a foot roller like the Foot Log or a tennis or golf ball to roll your foot over before getting out of bed. This will help to get blood flowing and loosen the plantar from sleeping overnight.
- Consider wearing a night splint to keep your foot in the dorsi-flexion position (i.e., foot is pulled back toward the shin instead of pointed), which prevents the plantar fascia from contracting.
- Cross-train with swimming and indoor cycling (avoid standing and riding outside on hills).
- Consider physical therapy or Active Release Technique treatment to help with exercises to stretch your calves and keep your muscles functioning properly.
- Consider seeing a podiatrist and having orthotics made to correct any imbalances in your lower extremities.

4. **Patella femoral pain syndrome:** Patella femoral pain syndrome is pain in front of the knee and usually caused by overuse, injury, or excessive weight or tracking of the knee cap. Here are some remedies you might want to consider:
   - RICE = Rest, Ice, Compression, and Elevation to reduce the immediate pain, but continue with icing daily and use anti-inflammatories to reduce the inflammation.
   - See a physical therapist to help you strengthen your hips and lower extremities like glutes, quads, and hamstrings to avoid this injury in the future.
   - Try taping just under the kneecap in an "X" fashion to reduce pressure on the tendon while it heals.
   - Improve your technique or position on the bike and running to ensure you have proper form to avoid injury.

5. **Morton's neuroma:** Morton's neuroma is an inflamed or swollen nerve in the ball of the foot usually between the third and fourth toes. It is usually a result of irritation, pressure, or injury and causes a burning or numbness sensation in the ball of your foot. It can be a result of overtraining or having an improper bike or running shoe fit or a bunion or some other injury. Here are some remedies you might want to consider:

- RICE = Rest, Ice, Compression, and Elevation to reduce the immediate pain, but continue with icing daily and use anti-inflammatories to reduce the inflammation.
- Get a wide-toe box sneaker or bike shoe or use thinner socks to give you extra room to allow your feet to spread. Use a flat shoe and avoid high-heeled shoes, as they can be the cause of the neuroma.
- Seek professional help where corticosteroid injections may be recommended or, as a last resort, surgery.

6. **Bacteria/yeast infections/cysts:** These are usually a result of positioning on the bike or bacteria built up in bike shorts or if a woman generally has that tendency. Here are some remedies you might want to consider:
   - Get a proper bike fit/adjust current bike position to avoid too much pressure on the soft tissue. Switching out your current bike seat for a more pro-woman-type seat might be in order.
   - Shower immediately after cycling to avoid infections.
   - Sterilize your cycling shorts regularly and generally keep that area clean and ventilated with loose cotton underwear.

7. **Other overuse injuries:** With a sport like triathlon where you spend many hours swimming, biking, and running, there is a tendency to develop overuse injuries. It can also be caused by an increase or doing too much exercise before your body has adjusted—the infamous "too much too soon!"—or biomechanical issues that manifest as you increase your volume, intensity, and durations. Here are some remedies you might want to consider:
   - RICE = Rest, Ice, Compression, and Elevation to reduce the immediate pain, but continue with icing daily and use anti-inflammatories to reduce the inflammation.
   - Cross-train with a nonimpact or weight-bearing exercise to avoid continuing injuring yourself.
   - See an ART (Active Release Technique) provider and a physical therapist to work on areas of weakness and develop and strengthen those areas.

• Work with a qualified coach who can help you plan your training around proper weekly, monthly, and annual cycles.

In summary, our health-related and physical injuries are what keep us from training as desired, performing at our best, and ultimately meeting our goals. The reality is that if we take a commonsense approach to our health by getting regular physicals, regular gynecological exams, and annual mammograms, we will have addressed 90 percent of our health issues. Align yourself with a health-care provider you are comfortable with and schedule your exams the same time every year, or twice a year where necessary. You would or should do this whether you are an athlete or not.

And lastly, the way you approach an injury will determine how quickly you recover and its reoccurrence. We say this to our athletes all the time: listen to your body and recognize the warning signs before an ache manifests itself into an injury. Rely on your own judgment and avoid plowing through a workout if you are injured, and always use your cross-training options, when possible. Recognize that every athlete, including yourself, is different and responds differently to exercise volumes, intensity, and durations. Know yourself, know your body, and you will have a great experience in this sport.

CHAPTER 16

Recovery and Maintenance Training

Optimism is the faith that leads to achievement. Nothing can be done without hope and confidence.

—Helen Keller

Congratulations! You have achieved your goal and raced a great race. Now what?

The programs in this book up until this point helped you to prepare for all of the popular triathlon race distances, from Sprint to Iron-Distance, so now we are going to talk about what types of training we should do after our races.

Triathletes can be extreme people and we see everything from the athlete who doesn't want to train after achieving her goal and wants to reward herself by putting her feet up for several weeks, to the athletes who are so excited and motivated after their race that they want to race the next weekend, if not the next day. In fact, neither of these extremes is optimal and both can be risky for your health.

We definitely need to keep moving. A sensible active recovery will allow your body to repair and revitalize itself and also retain its hard-earned fitness. As we like to say, our bodies need an opportunity to work the race out of our system. Too little activity will not allow this to happen as quickly and as completely, and jumping back into another race too quickly will only serve to break your body down more. Best case, you will probably have a flat racing performance. Worse case you may suffer an injury. We want to hit just the right level of activity for optimal fitness and health results.

Generally, there are two possible directions to head in after a race. Either we plan to go right back into training for another race as soon as our recovery phase has been completed, or we plan to transition into some type of off-season maintenance phase.

An IronFit Moment

Beware of the Post-Race Blues

After focusing so intensely on a great and worthy goal, many athletes feel a mental letdown in the weeks and months following their accomplishment. If this happens to you, don't worry, it happens to the best of us. We are goal-oriented people and when we don't have a goal, we can easily drift. This is why the best cure for the post-race blues is another worthy challenge. Set a new goal and commit to it. As soon as you do, everything will start to improve for the better. It's amazing how registering for a race can have such an impact. But for certain people—like us—it does.

It doesn't need to be as big a goal as your recent accomplishment. Any worthy goal will do. As long as you feel excited and motivated by it. The time frame is important too. Not too soon, but not too far away, either. For most athletes, something in the three- to six-month time frame works best.

In the following section we present three specific two-week training plans for the two weeks following your race. These plans correspond to the Competitive, Intermediate, and Just-Finish levels used throughout the training plans in this book. The plans all offer a flexible range of weekly hours. Generally, we suggest you gravitate more to the higher end of the range if you'd like to focus more on the longer-distance races and the lower end of the range if you gravitate more to shorter distance races.

The first of the two weeks is designed for a sensible recovery. It includes moderate fully aerobic training in each of the three sports and the durations gradually build back up. We like to think of this as a "reverse taper." Once completing this one week, the athlete may choose to then start the training plan for her next race.

If on the other hand, the athlete is planning not to race for at least a couple of months and instead transitioning into a maintenance phase, then the second of the two weeks serves as a model week for how she should train during her off-season.

Following are our suggested training programs for the two weeks after your triathlon for each of the Competitive, Intermediate, and Just-Finish athletes.

Competitive Athlete: Two-Week Recovery/Off-Season Maintenance Program (Note: Swims #1 through 6 can be found on pages 112 to 113):

COMPETITIVE PROGRAM — RECOVERY/OFF-SEASON MAINTENANCE

WEEK 1	SWIM	BIKE	RUN
M	#1—Opt.-easy	Rest day/slide day	Rest day/slide day
T	Off	Off	45 min. Z1—easy
W	#2	Trans: 45 min. Z1 to Z2 (QC)	15 min. Z1 to Z2
R	Off	45–60 min. Z1 to Z2	Off
F	#3	Off	45–60 min. Z1 to Z2
S	Off	1:00–1:15 hr. Z1 to Z2	Off
S	Off	Off	45–60 min. Z1 to Z2
Totals: 7:00–9:00 hr.	2:00–3:00 hr.	2:30–3:00 hr.	2:30–3:00 hr.

WEEK 2	SWIM	BIKE	RUN
M	#4—Opt.	Rest day/slide day	Rest day/slide day
T	Off	Off	60 min. Z2
W	#5	Trans: 45 min. Z2 (QC)	15–30 min. Z2
R	Off	45–60 min. Z2	Off
F	#6	Off	45–60 min. Z2
S	Off	1:30–2:15 hr. Z2	Off
S	Off	Opt: 60 min. Z1 (100+ rpm)	1:00–1:30 hr. Z1 to Z2
Totals: 8:00–12:00 hr.	2:00–3:00 hr.	3:00–5:00 hr.	3:00–4:00 hr.

Intermediate Athlete: Two-Week Recovery/Off-Season Maintenance Program (Note: Swims #45 through 48 can be found on page 115):

INTERMEDIATE PROGRAM — RECOVERY/OFF-SEASON MAINTENANCE

WEEK 1	SWIM	BIKE	RUN
M	Rest day/ slide day	Rest day/slide day	Rest day/slide day
T	#45	Off	30–45 min. Z1—easy
W	Off	Trans: 30 min. Z1 to Z2 (QC)	15 min. Z1 to Z2
R	#46	45 min. Z1 to Z2	Off
F	Rest day/ slide day	Rest day/slide day	Rest day/slide day
S	Off	45–75 min. Z1 to Z2	Off
S	Off	Off	45–60 min. Z1 to Z2
Totals: 5:00– 6:00 hr.	1:30 hr.	2:00–2:30 hr.	1:30–2:00 hr.

WEEK 2	SWIM	BIKE	RUN
M	Rest day/ slide day	Rest day/slide day	Rest day/slide day
T	#47	Off	45–60 min. Z2
W	Off	Trans: 45 min. Z2 (QC)	15 min. Z2
R	#48	45–60 min. Z2	Off
F	Rest day/ slide day	Rest day/slide day	Rest day/slide day
S	Off	1:00–2:00 hr. Z2	Off
S	Off	Off	1:00–1:30 hr. Z1 to Z2
Totals: 6:00– 8:00 hr.	1:30 hr.	2:30–3:45 hr.	2:00–2:45 hr.

Just-Finish Athlete: Two-Week Recovery/Off-Season Maintenance Program (Note: Swims #25 through 28 can be found on page 114):

JUST-FINISH PROGRAM — RECOVERY/OFF-SEASON MAINTENANCE

WEEK 1	SWIM	BIKE	RUN
M	Rest day/ slide day	Rest day/slide day	Rest day/slide day
T	#25	Off	30 min. Z1 easy
W	Off	Trans: 15 min. Z1 to Z2 (QC)	15 min. Z1 to Z2
R	#26	30 min. Z1 to Z2	Off
F	Rest day/ slide day	Rest day/slide day	Rest day/slide day
S	Off	30–60 min. Z1 to Z2	Off
S	Off	Off	30–60 min. Z1 to Z2
Totals: 4:00–5:00 hr.	1:30 hr.	1:15–1:45 hr.	1:15–1:45 hr.

WEEK 2	SWIM	BIKE	RUN
M	Rest day/ slide day	Rest day/slide day	Rest day/slide day
T	#27	Off	30–45 min. Z2
W	Off	Trans: 15–30 min. Z2 (QC)	15 min. Z2
R	#28	30–45 min. Z2	Off
F	Rest day/ slide day	Rest day/slide day	Rest day/slide day
S	Off	30–75 min. Z2	Off
S	Off	Off	30–60 min. Z1 to Z2
Totals: 4:00–6:00 hr.	1:30 hr.	1:15–2:30 hr.	1:15–2:00 hr.

Off-Season Training Focus

Through our years of coaching female triathletes, we have seen many who do not realize what a great opportunity the off-season presents. While some athletes prefer to "just get away from it for a while," others use this time wisely to prepare themselves to take their performances to the next level when they return to racing.

If you asked us for just one thing to focus on in the off-season, we would quickly say, "Improve your weakest link." Ultimately our triathlon performance is always going to be limited by our weakest sport. Ironically, most athletes tend to focus less on their weakest sport in the off-season and enjoy their time away from it. The problem with this approach is that when the next racing season comes around, your weakness is still your weakness and it will again hold you back just like it did before.

We see this most often in swimming, as we run a large local Masters Swimming program. Many of our triathletes who are weakest in the swim tend to disappear from Masters for a couple of months after the summer racing season, only to return a couple of months before the start of the next season. When they do return, we see that their swim has deteriorated, and it takes them a couple of months just to get back to the level they were at, let alone see any improvement.

What is extra discouraging is when they see their previous swim lane mates having moved up to the next fastest lane because they had been focusing on improving their swim over the off-season.

Our clear recommendation is to make your off-season goal to focus on your weakest link so much over the off-season that you enter the next racing season with that sport at its best level ever. Athletes who do this tend to see yearly overall triathlon performance gains, as well as greater long-term reward and enjoyment from the sport.

As we like to say, "Befriend the enemy." If you aren't that fond of swimming, don't just swim more often in the off-season, truly immerse yourself in it. We suggest things like swimming an extra session per week, taking swim technique lessons, focusing more on technique drills, and entering some Masters Swim meets. An exciting and motivating approach to this is to race a couple of the longer pool distances (e.g., 500 and 1,650 yards, or 400 and 1,500 meters). Then, consider those times your benchmarks to focus on improving during the off-season. Toward the end of the off-season, race these distances again and see how much you can beat them by.

Athletes who employ this off-season plan usually find that they not only see great improvements in their swim performance, but more important they enter the next triathlon season with newfound confidence and love for the sport.

While it is always tough to generalize, we tend to see cycling as the sport of the greatest potential improvement for women. This is, of course, not true across the board, but it is usually the area in which we can find the greatest off-season improvements.

If this seems true for you, consider an off-season focus on cycling, and in this case, strength work, like the strength and core programs in this book, can greatly contribute to this process.

But whatever your weakest link is, as we like to say, "Let's turn our weaknesses into strengths, and let's turn our strengths into weapons."

In addition to focusing on your weakest link, here are more suggestions for the off-season:

- **Endurance activity substitutions:** While we want to stick mostly with swimming, cycling, and running in the off-season, it is a great time to substitute in other comparable endurance sports activities for some of our bike and/or runs sessions. This can add variety and enjoyment to the off-season, while continuing to build and maintain your aerobic base. The best options for this include cross-country skiing, mountain biking, mountain climbing, and hiking.
- **Lifestyle changes:** Some athletes want to expand beyond just triathlon activities to lifestyle, relaxation, and spiritual endeavors as well. With a little less time needed for training, the off-season is a great time to start these. Popular activities along these lines are yoga, Pilates, mediation, breathing exercises, and other mixed training. If you can start one of these types of activities during the off-season, you will likely be able to develop some consistency with it, and then be able to keep up with it throughout the year.
- **Stay lean:** Many athletes mistakenly put on excess weight during the off-season. While a few pounds can easily be shaved off when you eventually go back into racing season, some athletes really let it slip and

put on a lot of weight. We are often amazed at how some athletes can put on 10 to 20 pounds or even more in the off-season. Please don't let this happen to you. It is not healthy and this weight cannot be safely taken off in a short period of time. The off-season is an important time to focus on your health and nutrition, and with more time to really focus on it, the off-season is a great time to establish new good habits that will continue throughout the year. Please consider our approaches and suggestions in Chapter 3 and stay lean and healthy year-round.

- **Functional Strength and Core Training:** The off-season is often a great time to focus on strength and core training. Since our overall swim, bike, and run training time is reduced, most athletes find they have a little more availability in their schedule for this important area. Focusing on functional strength and core training in the off-season will have you entering the next racing season stronger and more injury proof. The time-efficient functional strength and core program in Chapter 7 details exactly what you need to do in the off-season.

As we said at the start of this book, you are already part of the illustrious history of women in the sport of triathlon. That is something to be very proud of. We hope this book contributes to your success and enjoyment on your triathlon journey. Keep up the great work and we will see you at the finish line!

Acknowledgments

We wish to thank the following individuals: Kellie Brown, Maureen Cullen, Corey Debiasse, Breena Fishback, Judith Germano, Yvonne Hernandez, Marienne Hill-Treadway, Lynn Kellogg, Laura Litwin, James Mitchell, Beth Poore, Marcia Postillian, Francis Quinn, Heidi Sessner, Melissa Silverman, Karen Smyers, Aya Stevens, Scott Tinley, Debra Trebitz, and Keith Wallman.

Glossary

abs: Abdominal muscles.

Aerobic Energy System: An energy system that primarily uses oxygen and stored fat to power physical activity. This system can support activity for prolonged periods, as stored fat and oxygen are available in almost endless supply. Even a highly trained athlete with body-fat percentages in the single digits has more than enough stored fat for several ultradistance races back-to-back.

Anaerobic Energy System: An energy system that primarily uses glycogen (stored sugar) to power physical activity. This system can support activity for relatively short periods of time, as the body stores sugar in relatively small quantities.

basil metabolic rate (BMR): The number of calories needed to be consumed each day to allow our bodies to function normally and maintain current body weight.

body mass index (BMI): A relative measure of body height to body weight for purposes of determining a healthy or nonhealthy weight.

BOSU®Ball (acronym for both sides utilized): This is an inflated "half-ball" with a flat side and a half dome side. This popular piece of equipment is primarily used to develop balance and stability on an uneven and/or unstable surface.

brick session: See "transition session."

calorie: A basic unit of energy. Our bodies require energy to perform virtually all functions and get this energy in the form of calories. Carbohydrates and proteins have about 4 calories per gram, while fat has about 9 calories per gram.

carbohydrate loading: Various dietary approaches for the purpose of increasing glycogen stores prior to an endurance race.

cool down: A lower-intensity activity that helps the body to gradually and safely transition from a relatively higher-intensity activity.

core muscles: Includes abdominals, back, buttocks, pelvic floor, and hips.

dumbbells: Handheld exercise weights available in various coatings from plastic to metal and various weights from 1 pound to 50-plus pounds.

electrolytes: Common examples of electrolytes are sodium, potassium, chloride, and carbon dioxide. They are needed by our cells to function properly and keep the body's fluids in balance.

foam roller: This piece of exercise equipment is made of hard foam and is usually 36 inches long and 6 inches around, with varying densities used for self massage.

45-minute window: The time period of opportunity after a training session to jump-start the replenishment of glycogen stores.

fueling: Within the context of endurance sports, this term refers to the process of consuming calories before, during, and after training and racing to build and maintain high levels of energy and to boost recovery.

fueling logistics: The means by which athletes access their needed calories during competition.

glutes: Short for the gluteus maximus, medius, and minimus muscle group.

glycogen: The form in which the body stores sugar (carbohydrates) for the purpose of powering muscle activity.

hydrating: Within the context of endurance sports, this term refers to the process of drinking fluids before, during, and after training and racing to support optimal performance, safety, and good health.

hydration logistics: The means by which athletes access their needed fluids during competition.

kettle bells: These are handheld weights, but unlike dumbbells, the center of mass is extended beyond the hand. This facilitates ballistic and swinging movements. Like dumbbells, they are available in various coatings and weights.

lactate threshold: The heart rate level at which lactate begins to accumulate at a faster rate in the muscles than the body can clear.

medicine ball: This is a weighted ball with a rubberized or leather coating used in core and functional strength-training exercises. It is available in various weights from 1 to 20 pounds.

overload principle: According to the American Council on Exercise: "One of the principles of human performance that states that beneficial adaptations occur in response to demands applied to the body at levels beyond a certain threshold (overload), but within the limits of tolerance and safety."

quads: Short for the muscles of the quadriceps.

reps or repetitions: The number of times an exercise movement is repeated within an exercise set.

sets: A specific grouping of repetitions of a specific exercise movement. Typically, there will be one to three sets of each exercise within a specific exercise program.

75-Minute Fueling Guideline, The: The approximate point in a workout when water alone is not enough for most athletes to maintain the same performance level. Adequate calories, in addition to hydration, are needed.

stability ball (aka Swiss ball): This inflated exercise ball is the most popular and widely used piece of core-training equipment. It is important that it is properly sized to fit your height.

stretch cords and resistance tubing: These are rubber or plastic cords, usually with handles and available in various resistances.

Sweat Rate Test: A physical test performed by an athlete to help determine his or her hydration needs while training and racing.

taper phase: A pre-race training period of decreasing training volume for the purpose of having the athlete rested and energized for competition.

T1: The transition between the swim and cycling phases of a triathlon.

training volume: The combination of training duration, frequency, and intensity.

transition session (aka brick session): A training session that involves two sports separated by a brief period for the athlete to change from the clothing and equipment of one sport to that of the other.

T2: The transition between the cycling and running phases of a triathlon.

VO2Max: A measure of an athlete's ability to process oxygen and convert it to energy.

warm-up: A movement routine that prepares the athlete's body for training or racing by raising his or her core body temperature and lubricating joints and tendons.

watts-based training: A training approach for cycling that involves measuring intensity by produced wattage.

Suggested Reading

The books listed here have been very helpful to us over the years and have provided a great deal of information to us as we compiled our research for this book. They may prove useful to you as well.

Be Iron Fit: Time-Efficient Training Secrets for Ultimate Fitness. 2nd edition. Don Fink. Lyons Press. 2010.

The Big Book of Endurance Training and Racing. Philip Maffetone and Mark Allen. Skyhorse Publishing. 2010.

Core Performance Endurance. Mark Verstegen and Pete Williams. Rodale Inc. 2007.

Endurance Sports Nutrition, Strategies for Training, Racing, and Recovery. 2nd edition. Suzanne Girard Eberle, MS, RD. Human Kinetics. 2007.

Exercising through Your Pregnancy. 2nd edition. James F. Clapp, III, M.D. and Catherine Clam, M.S. Addicus Books, 2012.

Heart Rate Training. Roy Benson and Declan Connolly. Human Kinetics. 2011.

Instant Relief: Tell Me Where It Hurts and I'll Tell You What to Do. Peggy Brill and Susan Suffes. Bantam. 2007.

IronFit Strength Training and Nutrition for Endurance Athletes. Don Fink and Melanie Fink. Lyons Press. 2013.

Lifestyle and Weight Management Consultant Manual. Richard T. Cotton. American Council on Exercise. 1996.

Mastering the Marathon: Time-Efficient Training Secrets for the 40-plus Athlete. Don Fink. Lyons Press. 2010.

Personal Trainer Manual—The Resource for Fitness Professionals. Richard T. Cotton. American Council on Exercise. 1997.

Program Design for Personal Trainers: Bridging Theory into Application. Douglas S. Brooks, MS. Human Kinetics. 1997.

Sports Nutrition for Endurance Athletes. 2nd edition. Monique Ryan, MS, RD, LDN. Velo Press. 2007.

Training Lactate Pulse-Rate. Peter G. J. M. Janssen. Polar Electro Oy. 1987.

The Triathlete's Training Bible. Joe Friel. Velo Press. 2009.

Triathlon for Every Woman. Meredith Atwood. Tricycle Books. 2012.

Triathlon for Girls Like Us. Gloria Safar. Create Space Independent. 2010.

Triathlon Science. Joe Friel and Jim Vance. Human Kinetics. 2013.

Triathlons for Women. Sally Edwards. Velo Press. 2010.

The Woman Triathlete. Christina Gandolfo. Human Kinetics. 2004.

Suggested Websites

Active Release Technique: activerelease.com

American Council on Exercise: acefitness.org

British Triathlon: britishtriathlon.org

Debra Trebitz: debratrebitzphotography.com

Esprit de She: espritdeshe.com

IronFit: ironfit.com

Iron Girl: irongirl.com

James Mitchell Photography: jamesmitchell.eu

Jersey Girl Triathlon: jerseygirltriathlon.com

Lose It: loseit.com

My Fitness Pal: myfitnesspal.com

Triathlon Australia: www.triathlon.org.au

Triathlon Canada: triathloncanada.com

Triathlon New Zealand: www.triathlon.org.nz

Tri Find: trifind.com

Tri Goddess Triathlon: epicraces.com

Tri Life Photos: trilifephotos.com

USA Triathlon: usatriathlon.org

US Masters Swimming: usms.org

Weight Watchers: weightwatchers.com

Yvonne Hernandez: bbasports.com

Index

About the Authors

Don Fink is an internationally known triathlon and running coach/trainer and author of the popular endurance-sports training books *Be Iron Fit: Time-Efficient Training Secrets for Ultimate Fitness* (2004), *Be Iron Fit, second edition* (2010), *Mastering the Marathon: Time-Efficient Training Secrets for the 40-Plus Athlete* (2010), *IronFit Strength Training and Nutrition for Endurance Athletes* (2013), and *IronFit Secrets for Half Iron-Distance Triathlon Success* (2013), all published by Globe Pequot Press. Among his credentials, Don is a

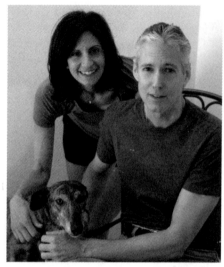

Don Fink, Melanie Fink, and Sheena
Lynn Kellogg/www.trilifephotos.com

Certified Personal Trainer by the American Council on Exercise (ACE) and he is a Professional Member of the National Strength and Conditioning Association (NSCA). Don and his wife, Melanie, train endurance athletes on five continents through their business, IronFit (IronFit.com). Don and Melanie have utilized their innovative approaches to coach hundreds of athletes to personal best times and breakthrough performances in triathlon, the marathon, and other sports.

In addition to being an endurance sports coach/trainer, Don Fink is an elite athlete. He has raced over thirty Ironman triathlons (2.4-mile swim, 112-mile bike, and 26.2-mile run) and has many age-group victories and course records to his credit. Don's time of 9:08 at the 2004 Ironman Florida is one of the fastest times ever recorded by an athlete in the 45–49 age group.

Don Fink also placed in the top three overall in the 2002 Ultra Man World Championships (6.2-mile swim, 270-mile bike, and 52.4-mile run) on the Big Island of Hawaii.

Melanie's credentials include Certified Personal Trainer by the American Council on Exercise (ACE) and a Regional Council Member of USA Triathlon Mid-Atlantic. Melanie co-authored the popular endurance sports training book *IronFit Strength Training: Nutrition for Endurance Athletes* (2013) and *IronFit Secrets for Half Iron-Distance Triathlon Success* (2013). In addition to being a sports coach/trainer and Masters Swimming coach, Melanie Fink is an elite athlete. She has many age-group and overall victories in triathlon and open-water swimming competitions, has completed twelve Iron-distance triathlons (including the Hawaii Ironman twice), and completed Ultra Man Canada (6.2-mile swim, 270-mile bike, and 52.4-mile run) in Penticton, British Columbia. Melanie's passion is helping women to get into the sport of triathlon and to become athletes for life.

Don and Melanie Fink live in Carroll County, New Hampshire.